Manual of Structural Kinesiology

Clem W. Thompson Ph.D., F.A.C.S.M.
(deceased)

Clem W. Thompson Ph.D., F.A.C.S.M.
(deceased)
Professor Physical Education, Emeritus
Mankato State University
Mankato, Minnesota

R. T. Floyd M.A.T., A.T.,C.
Associate Professor of Physical Education and Athletic Training
The University of West Alabama
Livingston, Alabama

TWELFTH EDITION

with **312** illustrations

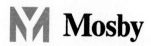

M Mosby

St. Louis Baltimore Boston Chicago London Madrid Philadelphia Sydney Toronto

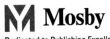
Mosby
Dedicated to Publishing Excellence

Editor-in-Chief: James M. Smith
Acquisitions Editor: Vicki Malinee
Developmental Editor: Amy K. Winston
Project Manager: Gayle May Morris
Production Editor: Mary Cusick Drone
Manufacturing Supervisor: Kathy Grone
Designer: Susan Lane
Cover Design: GW Graphics
Cover Photo: © Duomo/Steven E. Sutton

The author and publisher disclaim any responsibility for any adverse effects or consequences from the misapplication or injudicious use of information contained within this text.

Printed in the United States of America
Composition by Graphic World, Inc.
Printing/binding by Custom Printing Company

Mosby–Year Book, Inc.
11830 Westline Industrial Drive
St. Louis, Missouri 63146

Library of Congress Cataloging-in-Publication Data

Thompson, Clem W.
    Manual of structural kinesiology / Clem W. Thompson, R.T. Floyd.
 - 12th ed.
        p.   cm.
    Includes index.
    ISBN 0-8016-7831-5
    1. Kinesiology.   2. Muscles.   I. Floyd, R. T.   II. Title.
QP303.T58   1993
612.7′6—dc20   93-23382
                                                              CIP

96 97 / 9 8 7 6 5 4 3 2

613.71
(Tho)

Manual of Structural Kinesiology

1 Week Loan

This book is due for return on or before the last date shown below

1 9 APR 2010		

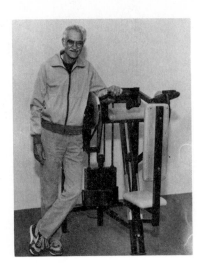

Mosby–Year Book mourns the death in 1990 of Clem W. Thompson, Ph.D., F.A.C.S.M., whose career achievements and enthusiasm for physical fitness helped to shape the field of physical education for his students and colleagues alike. Dr. Thompson authored the fourth through the eleventh editions of this highly successful textbook, *Manual of Structural Kinesiology*. He published many research papers, articles, and presentations; but he considered this book to be his most important professional accomplishment.

Dr. Thompson was a professor emeritus of physical education at Mankato State University in Mankato, Minnesota, where he served on the faculty for 25 years. He had taught at the University of Arkansas and Boston University before coming to MSU and retired from teaching in 1984. Dr. Thompson was a member of The American Alliance for Health, Physical Education, Recreation and Dance and served on various governing boards of the American Heart Association.

Dr. Thompson received his undergraduate degree from Knox College in Galesburg, Illinois in 1938, his master's degree from the University of Illinois in 1941, and his doctorate from the University of Iowa in 1950.

Dr. Thompson was a pioneer in the campaign against smoking when it was more popular to smoke than to denounce it. He was a leader in the efforts to awaken Americans to the need to be healthy. His own outstanding personal example of physical fitness touched the lives of thousands of students and hundreds of his colleagues. His legacy of a commitment to a fit and healthy life will be perpetuated in the professional careers of them all.

To
my son
Robert Thomas
and my daughter
Rebecca

R.T.F.

Preface

Revising this text has been both a challenging and enjoyable experience. I have long been impressed with the approach that the late Dr. Clem Thompson used in presenting this material. First being exposed to this book as an undergraduate and then using several editions in my teachings, I have become very familiar with the style of the text and have developed further insight into how students use the information as they learn.

I agree with Dr. Thompson in attributing the continued strength and popularity of this book to the clear, concise, and simplistic presentation. Because of my respect for his work and its effectiveness, I have tried to preserve his approach while supplementing it with applicable information and insight collected throughout my career thus far.

This text, first published in 1948, has undergone many positive changes over the last 45 years. My goals have been to make this revision as applicable as possible to everyday physical activity and to make it more understandable and easier to use for the student. I have tried to improve the consistency of the presentation order so that the reader can concentrate on the material and not be distracted by changing formats. I challenge kinesiology students while reading to immediately apply the content of this text to physical activities with which they are individually familiar. I hope that the student will simultaneously palpate his or her own moving joints and contracting muscles while reading to gain application. I believe strongly that through practical laboratory application the student will not only gain a better understanding of the concepts but will retain them more for future use, which is really our ultimate goal.

Audience

Applied kinesiologists, athletic trainers, athletic coaches, physical educators, physical therapists, health club instructors, strength and conditioning specialists, and others who are responsible for improving and maintaining the muscular strength and endurance of individuals will benefit from this text.

With the tremendous growth in the number of participants in an ever increasing spectrum of physical activity, it is imperative that medical, health, and education professionals involved in providing instruction and information to the physically active be correct and accountable for the teachings that they provide. The variety of exercise machines, techniques, strengthening programs, and training programs is constantly expanding and changing, but the musculoskeletal system is constant in its design and architecture. Regardless of the goals sought or the approaches used in exercise activity, the human body is the basic ingredient and must be thoroughly understood and considered to maximize performance capabilities and minimize undesirable results. Most advances in exercise science continue to result from a better understanding of the body and how it functions. I believe that an individual in this field can never learn enough about structure and function of the human body.

Those who are charged with the responsibility of providing instruction to the physically active will find this text a helpful and valuable resource in their hopefully never-ending quest for knowledge and understanding of human movement.

New to this Edition

Major changes to this edition include the addition of pronunciations and nervous innervations for each muscle. I have renamed the former observation and exercise sections as functional application and strengthening. This new section is now provided for every muscle on an individual basis. The content under each has been expanded to include more emphasis on modern applications of the role of the muscle in exercise activities. The relationship between the muscle and related injuries is also often addressed, and specific simple strengthening exercises are listed for each muscle.

In the eight chapters that address specific body parts, photographs are included that depict each movement of the body part. Joint classifications and ranges of motion have been added for consistency. Several muscles have been added, and muscle analysis charts have either been expanded or added. Several illustrations have been added, along with the inclusion of separate illustrations detailing the origin and insertion of practically every muscle discussed. The student objectives have been revised when appropriate to reflect changes, and several new references have been added to reflect more current resources. Some revision of the laboratory and review exercises at the end of each chapter has taken place. Chapter 1, Foundations of Structural Kinesiology, has been expanded significantly to include more terminology with concise definitions that will hopefully remove some confusion from the student's mind during application.

One chapter from the previous edition has been expanded and divided to form Chapter 4, The Elbow and Radioulnar Joints, and Chapter 5, The Wrist and Hand Joints.

In Chapter 6, Muscular Analysis of Upper Extremities, I have attempted to clarify the terminology regarding muscular contractions. In Chapter 11, Muscular Analysis of Selected Exercises and Activities, there is a new section on muscular analysis, along with an expanded section on conditioning principles. Some of the exercise analyses have also been revised.

Chapter 12, Some Factors Affecting Motion and Movement, has been revised to provide more examples and applications along with its expanded terminology.

In addition, the Glossary has doubled in size to include the new material.

Acknowledgments

I initially became involved with this revision by request from Mosby to review the eleventh edition for suggested changes. During that time period five other active, current university instructors of kinesiology were selected by the publisher to review this text. Their many comments, ideas, and suggestions have served as an extremely helpful guide in this revision, and I am most grateful. These reviewers are:

Diane Arnold, N.A.
Foothill College

Dianne Busch, Ed.D.
Southwestern Oklahoma State University

Christine Stopka, Ph.D.
The University of Florida

James Whitehead, Ed.D.
The University of North Dakota

Carole Zebas, P.E.D.
The University of Kansas

I would also like to especially thank Gordon L. Graham, P.T., M.S., A.T.,C. of Mankato State University and Carole J. Zebas, P.E.D. of The University of Kansas for their review of my manuscript throughout this revision. They have provided much needed input and suggestions that have helped tremendously. I also acknowledge Mr. John Hood and Mrs. Linda Kimbrough of Birmingham, Alabama for the fine photographs and superb illustrations, respectively; Mr. Marcus Shapiro, who served as the model for the photographs; my typist, Mrs. Natalie Jeffcoat; my close personal friends who have provided a great deal of encouragement and support; and my colleagues at Livingston University—Mr. Brad Montgomery, Mrs. Mary Tew Long, and Dr. Billy Slay and at The University of Alabama—Dr. Mark Richardson, Dr. Ken Wright, and Ms. Lou Fincher—for their advice, suggestions, and support. My thanks also go to Amy Winston, Cheryl Gelfand-Grant, Vicki Malinee, and Mary Drone of the Mosby staff who have been most helpful in their assistance and suggestions in preparing the manuscript for publication.

R.T. Floyd

Contents

Foundations of structural kinesiology

Objectives

* To review the anatomy of the skeletal and muscle systems.

* To review and understand the terminology used to describe joint movements and body part locations.

* To review the planes of motion in relation to human movement.

* To describe and understand the various types of joints in the human body and their characteristics.

* To describe and demonstrate the joint movements.

Structural kinesiology is the study of muscles as they are involved in the science of movement. Both skeletal and muscular structures are involved. Bones are different sizes and shapes—particularly at the joints, which allow or limit the movements. Muscles vary greatly in size, shape, and structure from one part of the body to another.

More than 600 muscles are found in the human body. Most people who use this book do not need to know about each muscle. A majority of the muscles in the human body are small muscles located in the hands, feet, and spinal column. Anatomists, coaches, nurses, physical educators, physical therapists, physicians, athletic trainers, and others in health-related fields should have an adequate knowledge and understanding of all the large muscle groups so they can teach others how to strengthen, improve, and maintain these parts of the human body. This knowledge forms the basis of the exercise programs that should be followed to strengthen and maintain all of the muscles. In most cases, exercises that involve the larger primary movers also involve the smaller muscles.

Fewer than 100 of the largest and most important muscles, primary movers, are considered in this text. Other small muscles in the human body such as the multifidus, plantaris, scalenus, serratus posterior, and subclavius—are omitted, since they are exercised with other larger primary movers. In addition, most small muscles of the hand, feet, and spinal column are not considered.

Kinesiology students are frequently unable to see the forest through the trees: they become so engrossed in learning individual muscles that they lose sight of the total muscular system. They miss the "big picture"—that muscle groups move joints in given movements necessary for bodily movement and skilled performance.

Skeletal and muscular systems

Fig. 1-1 shows anterior and posterior views of the skeletal system. Two hundred and six bones make up the skeletal system, which provides support and protection for other systems of the body and provides for attachments of the muscles to the bones by which movement is produced.

Most students who take this course will have had a course in human anatomy, but a brief review is desirable before beginning the study of kinesiology. Other chapters provide additional information and more detailed illustrations of specific bones.

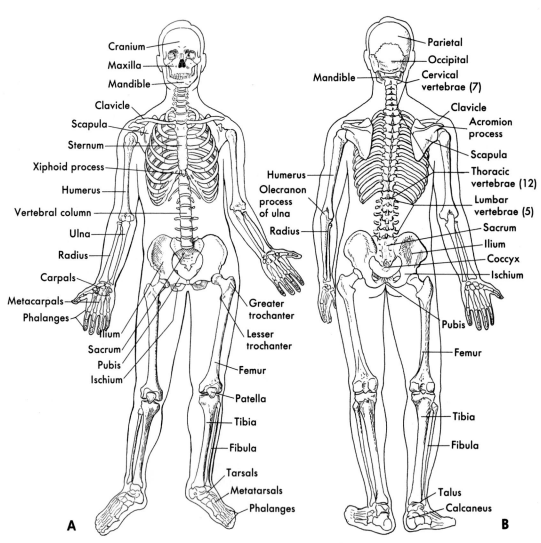

FIG. 1-1 • Skeleton. **A,** Anterior view; **B,** posterier view.

The total superficial muscular system is shown in Figs. 1-2 and 1-3. Any figure is limited, since many muscles are not surface muscles. Still, these figures will help provide a better overview of the entire superficial muscular structure.

Muscles shown in these figures, and many other muscles, are studied in more detail as each joint of the body is considered in other chapters of the book.

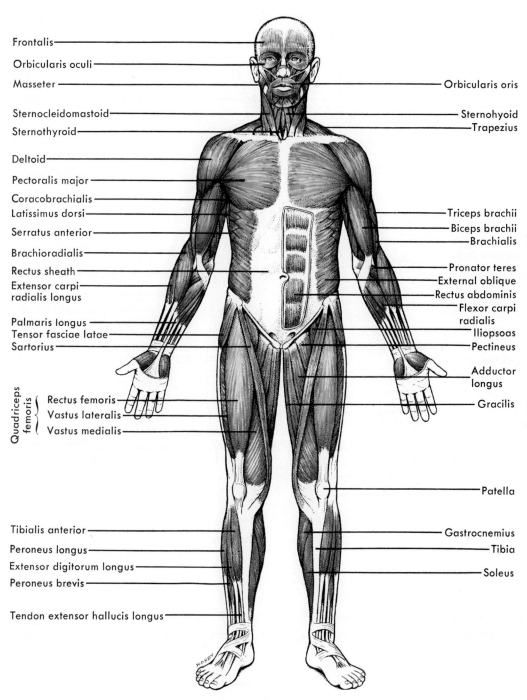

Frontalis
Orbicularis oculi
Masseter
Sternocleidomastoid
Sternothyroid
Deltoid
Pectoralis major
Coracobrachialis
Latissimus dorsi
Serratus anterior
Brachioradialis
Rectus sheath
Extensor carpi radialis longus
Palmaris longus
Tensor fasciae latae
Sartorius
Quadriceps femoris { Rectus femoris Vastus lateralis Vastus medialis
Tibialis anterior
Peroneus longus
Extensor digitorum longus
Peroneus brevis
Tendon extensor hallucis longus

Orbicularis oris
Sternohyoid
Trapezius
Triceps brachii
Biceps brachii
Brachialis
Pronator teres
External oblique
Rectus abdominis
Flexor carpi radialis
Iliopsoas
Pectineus
Adductor longus
Gracilis
Patella
Gastrocnemius
Tibia
Soleus

FIG. 1-2 • Muscles of the human body, anterior view.

From Thibodeau GA: Anatomy and physiology, St. Louis, 1987, Mosby.

FIG. 1-3 • Muscles of the human body, posterior view.

From Thibodeau GA: Anatomy and physiology, St. Louis, 1987, Mosby.

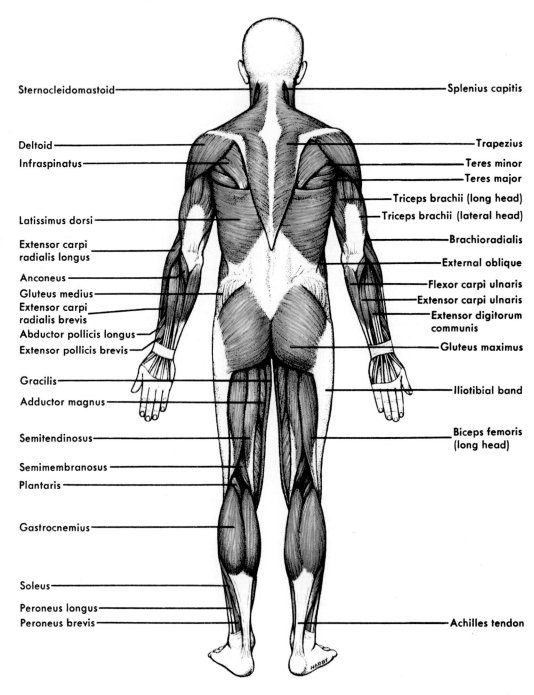

Sternocleidomastoid

Deltoid
Infraspinatus

Latissimus dorsi

Extensor carpi
radialis longus

Anconeus
Gluteus medius
Extensor carpi
radialis brevis

Abductor pollicis longus
Extensor pollicis brevis

Gracilis

Adductor magnus

Semitendinosus

Semimembranosus

Plantaris

Gastrocnemius

Soleus

Peroneus longus
Peroneus brevis

Splenius capitis

Trapezius
Teres minor
Teres major
Triceps brachii (long head)
Triceps brachii (lateral head)
Brachioradialis
External oblique
Flexor carpi ulnaris
Extensor carpi ulnaris
Extensor digitorum
communis
Gluteus maximus

Iliotibial band

Biceps femoris
(long head)

Achilles tendon

Anatomical directional terminology

FIG. 1-4

Anterior
in front or in the front part.

Anteroinferior
in front and below.

Anterolateral
in front and to the side, especially the outside.

Anteromedial
in front and toward the inner side or midline.

Anteroposterior
relating to both front and rear.

Anterosuperior
in front and above.

Contralateral
pertaining or relating to the opposite side.

Distal
situated away from the center or midline of the body, or from the point of origin.

Dorsal
relating to the back, posterior.

Inferior
(infra) below in relation to another structure, caudal.

Ipsilateral
on the same side.

Lateral
on or to the side, outside, farther from the median or midsagittal plane.

Medial
relating to the middle or center, nearer to the medial or midsagittal plane.

Posterior
behind, in back, or in the rear.

Posteroinferior
behind and below, in back and below.

Posterolateral
behind and to one side, specifically to the outside.

Posteromedial
behind and to the inner side.

Posterosuperior
situated behind and at the upper part.

Prone
the body lying face downward, stomach lying.

Proximal
nearest the trunk or the point of origin.

Superior
(supra) above in relation to another structure, higher, cephallic.

Supine
lying on the back, face upward position of the body.

Ventral
relating to the belly or abdomen.

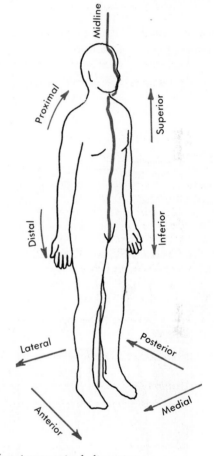

FIG. 1-4 • Anatomical directions.

From Arnheim DD: Modern principles of athletic training, ed 8, St. Louis, 1993, Mosby.

Planes of motion FIG. 1-5

When studying the various joints of the body and analyzing their movements, it is helpful to characterize them according to specific planes of motion.

There are three specific planes of motion in which the various joint movements can be classified. As movement occurs in a plane, the joint moves or turns about an axis that has a 90-degree relationship to that plane. Although each specific joint movement can be classified as being in one of the three planes of motion, our movements are usually not totally in one specific plane but occur as a combination of motions from more than one plane. These movements from the combined planes may be described as occurring in diagonal or oblique planes of motion.

Anteroposterior or sagittal plane

The anteroposterior or AP plane bisects the body from front to back, dividing it into right and left symmetrical halves. Generally, flexion and extension movements such as biceps curls, knee extensions, and sit-ups occur in this plane.

Lateral or frontal plane

The lateral plane, also known as the frontal or coronal plane, bisects the body laterally from side to side, dividing it into front and back halves. Abduction and adduction movements such as hip and shoulder abduction and spinal lateral flexion occur in this plane.

Transverse or horizontal plane

The transverse plane divides the body horizontally into superior and inferior halves. Generally, rotational movements such as pronation, supination, and spinal rotation occur in this plane.

FIG. 1-5 • Planes of motion.

Modified from Booher JM Thibodeau GA: Athletic injury assessment, ed 2, St. Louis, 1989, Mosby.

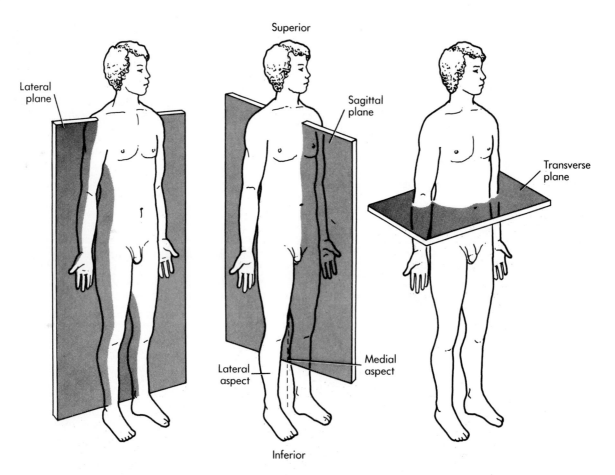

Types of joints

The articulation of two or more bones allows various types of movements. The extent and type of movement determines the name applied to the joint. Bone structure limits the kind and amount of movements in each joint. Some joints are very limited, whereas others have a variety of movement ranges. The type and range of movements are similar in all humans; but the freedom, range, and vigor of movements are limited by ligaments and muscles.

The articulations are grouped in three classes on the basis of the amount of movement possible.

Synarthrodial (immovable) joints (Fig. 1-6)
Found in the sutures of the cranial bones and sockets of the teeth.

Amphiarthrodial (slightly movable) joints (Fig. 1-7)
Structurally these articulations are divided into two groups:

Syndesmosis
Type of joint held together by strong ligamentous structures that allow minimal movement between the bones. Examples are the coracoclavicular joint and the inferior tibiofibular joint.

Synchondrosis
Type of joint separated by a fibrocartilage that allows very slight movement between the bones. Examples are the symphysis pubis and the costochondral joints of the ribs with the sternum.

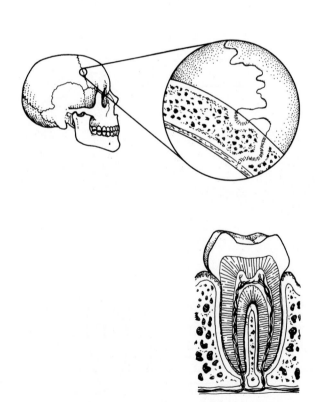

FIG. 1-6 • Synarthrodial joints.

Modified from Booher JM Thibodeau GA: Athletic injury assessment, ed 2, St. Louis, 1989, Mosby.

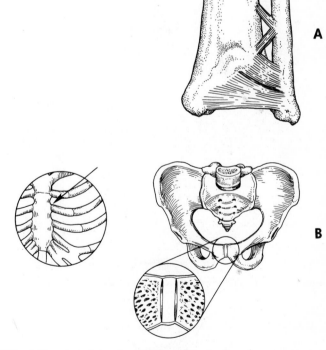

FIG. 1-7 • Amphiarthrodial joints. **A,** Syndesmosis joint; **B,** synchondrosis joint.

Modified from Booher JM Thibodeau GA: Athletic injury assessment, ed 2, St. Louis, 1989, Mosby.

Diarthrodial (freely movable) joints (Fig. 1-8)

Structurally this type of articulation can be divided into six groups:

Arthrodial (gliding joint)

Two plane or flat bony surfaces that butt against each other, permitting limited gliding movement. Examples are the carpal bones of the wrist and the tarsometatarsal joints in the foot.

Condyloidal (biaxial ball and socket joint)

Type of joint in which the bones permit movement in two planes without rotation. Examples are the wrist between the radius and the proximal row of the carpal bones or the second, third, fourth, and fifth metacarpophalangeal joints.

Enarthrodial (multiaxial ball and socket joint)

Type of joint that permits movement in all planes. Examples are the shoulder (glenohumeral) and hip joints.

Ginglymus (hinge joint)

Type of joint that permits a wide range of movement in only one plane. Examples are the elbow, ankle, and knee joints.

Sellar (saddle joint)

This type of reciprocal reception is found only in the thumb at the carpometacarpal joint and permits ball and socket movement with the exception of rotation.

Trochoidal (pivot joint)

Type of joint with a rotational movement around a long axis. An example is the rotation of the radius at the radioulnar joint.

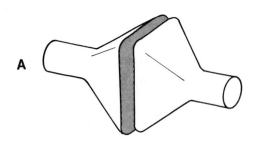

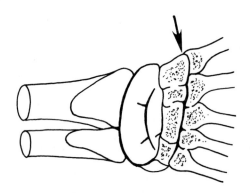

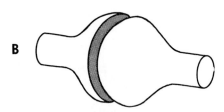

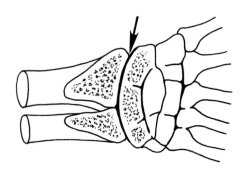

FIG. 1-8 • Diarthrodial joints. **A**, Arthrodial joint; **B**, condyloid joint.

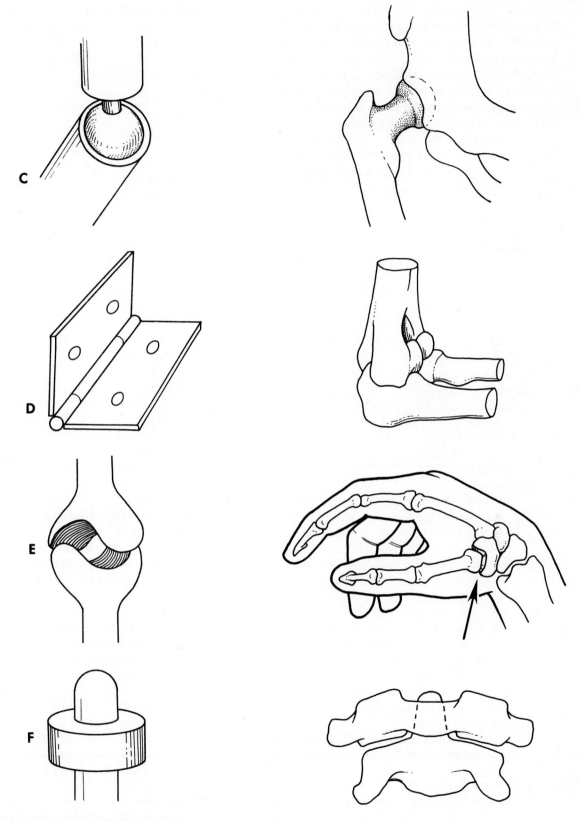

FIG. 1-8 cont'd • **C**, Enarthrodial joint; **D**, ginglymus joint; **E**, sellar joint; **F**, trochoidal joint.

Modified from Booher JM Thibodeau GA: Athletic injury assessment, ed 2, St. Louis, 1989, Mosby.

Movements in joints

In many joints, several different movements are possible. Some joints permit only flexion and extension; others permit a wide range of movements, depending largely on the joint structure.

Some movement terms may be used to describe motion at several joints throughout the body, whereas other terms are relatively specific to a joint or group of joints. Rather than list the terms alphabetically, we have chosen to group them according to the body area and pair them with opposite terms where applicable.

GENERAL

Abduction
Lateral movement away from the midline of the trunk. An example is raising the arms or legs to the side horizontally.

Adduction
Movement medially toward the midline of the trunk. An example is lowering the arms to the side or legs back to the anatomical position.

Flexion
Bending movement that results in a decrease of the angle in a joint by bringing bones together. An example is the elbow joint when the hand is drawn to the shoulder.

Extension
Straightening movement that results in an increase of the angle in a joint by moving bones apart. An example is when the hand moves away from shoulder.

Circumduction
Circular movement of a limb that describes a cone, combining the movements of flexion, extension, abduction, and adduction. An example is when the shoulder joint and the hip joint move in a circular fashion around a fixed point.

Diagonal abduction
Movement by a limb through a diagonal plane away from the midline of the body.

Diagonal adduction
Movement by a limb through a diagonal plane toward and across the midline of the body.

External rotation
Rotary movement around the longitudinal axis of a bone away from the midline of the body. Also known as rotation laterally, outward rotation, and lateral rotation.

Internal rotation
Rotary movement around the longitudinal axis of a bone toward the midline of the body. Also known as rotation medially, inward rotation, and medial rotation.

ANKLE AND FOOT

Eversion
Turning the sole of the foot outward or laterally. An example is standing with the weight on inner edge of the foot.

Inversion
Turning the sole of the foot inward or medially. An example is standing with the weight on outer edge of the foot.

Dorsal flexion
Flexion movement of the ankle that results in the top of foot moving toward the anterior tibia bone.

Plantar flexion
Extension movement of the ankle that results in the foot and or toes moving away from the body.

RADIOULNAR JOINT

Pronation
Internally rotating the radius where it lies diagonally across the ulna, resulting in the palm-down position of the forearm.

Supination
Externally rotating the radius where it lies parallel to the ulna, resulting in the palm-up position of the forearm.

SHOULDER GIRDLE AND SHOULDER JOINT

Depression
Inferior movement of the shoulder girdle. An example is returning to the normal position from a shoulder shrug.

Elevation
Superior movement of the shoulder girdle. An example is shrugging the shoulders.

Horizontal abduction
Movement of the humerus in the horizontal plane away from the midline of the body. Also known as horizontal extension or transverse abduction.

Horizontal adduction
Movement of the humerus in the horizontal plane toward the midline of the body. Also known as horizontal flexion or transverse adduction.

Protraction
Forward movement of the shoulder girdle away from the spine. Abduction of the scapula.

Retraction

Backward movement of the shoulder girdle toward the spine. Adduction of the scapula.

Rotation downward

Rotary movement of the scapula with the inferior angle of the scapula moving medially and downward.

Rotation upward

Rotary movement of the scapula with the inferior angle of the scapula moving laterally and upward.

SPINE

Lateral flexion (side bending)

Movement of the head and or trunk laterally away from the midline. Abduction of the spine.

Reduction

Return of the spinal column to the anatomic position from lateral flexion. Adduction of the spine.

WRIST and HAND

Radial flexion (radial deviation)

Abduction movement at the wrist of the thumb side of the hand toward the forearm.

Ulnar flexion (ulnar deviation)

Adduction movement at the wrist of the little finger side of the hand toward the forearm.

Opposition of the thumb

Diagonal movement of the thumb across palmar surface of the hand to make contact with the fingers.

These movements are considered in detail in the chapters to follow as they apply to the individual joints.

Combinations of movements can occur. Flexion or extension can occur with abduction or adduction.

Muscle terminology

Muscle contraction produces the force that causes joint movement in the human body. It is necessary to understand certain terms as body movement is considered.

The terms most commonly used are *origin* and *insertion*. It can be said that a muscle starts on one bone and ends on another bone. The origin of a muscle is considered the least movable part or the part that attaches closest to the midline or center of the body. The origin is known as the *proximal attachment*. The insertion is considered the most movable part or the part that attaches farthest from the midline or center of the body. The insertion is known as the *distal attachment*. For example, the biceps brachii muscle in the arm has its origin (least movable bone) on the scapula and its insertion (most movable bone) on the ulna. In some movements this process can be reversed. The specific joint chapters that follow explain this phenomenon in more detail. For each muscle studied, the origin and insertion are indicated.

All muscle contractions can be classified as being either *isometric* or *isotonic*. An isometric contraction occurs when tension is developed within the muscle but no appreciable change occurs in the joint angle or the length of the muscle. Isometric contractions may be thought of as *static* contractions because a significant amount of tension may be developed in the muscle to maintain the joint angle in a relatively static or stable position.

Isotonic contractions occur when tension is developed in the muscle while it either shortens or lengthens. Isotonic contractions are thought of as *dynamic* contractions because the varying degrees of tension in the muscle are causing the joint angles to change. The isotonic type of muscle contraction is classified further as being either *concentric* or *eccentric* on the basis of whether shortening or lengthening occurs.

Concentric contractions involve the muscle developing tension as it shortens. These contractions occur when the muscle develops enough force to overcome the applied resistance. The muscle may be thought of as causing movement against gravity or resistance. Concentric contractions are described as positive contractions.

Eccentric contractions involve the muscle lengthening under tension. These contractions occur when the muscle gradually lessens in tension to control the descent of the resistance. The weight or resistance may be thought of as overcoming the muscle contraction but not to the point that the muscle cannot control the descending movement. Eccentric contractions control movement with gravity or resistance and are described as negative contractions.

Worksheet exercises

As an aid to learning, for in-class or out-of-class assignments, or for testing, tearout worksheets are found at the end of the text (see pp. 213 and 214).

Posterior skeletal worksheet (no. 1)

On the posterior skeletal worksheet, list the names of the bones and all of the prominent features of each bone.

Anterior skeletal worksheet (no. 2)

On the anterior skeletal worksheet, list the names of the bones and all of the prominent features of each bone.

Laboratory and review exercises

1. Observe on a fellow student some of the muscles found in Figs. 1-2 and 1-3.
2. Locate the various types of joints on a human skeleton and palpate their movements on a living subject.
3. Individually practice the various joint movements, on yourself or with another subject.
4. Pick several different locations at random on your body and specifically describe these locations, using the correct anatomical directional terminology.
5. Complete the chart at the right by:
   a. Filling in the type of diarthrodial joint
   b. Listing the movements of the joint under the plane of motion in which they occur

References

Anthony C, Thibodeau G: Textbook of anatomy and physiology, ed 10, 1979, St. Louis, 1979, Mosby.

Goss CM: Gray's anatomy of the human body, ed 29, Philadelphia, 1973, Lea & Febiger.

Stedman TL: Stedman's medical dictionary, ed 23, Baltimore, 1976, Williams & Wilkins.

Steindler A: Kinesiology of the human body, Springfield, Ill, 1970, Charles C Thomas.

Joint type, movement, and plane of motion chart

Joint	Type	Plane of motions		
		Sagittal	Lateral	Transverse
Shoulder girdle				
Shoulder joint				
Elbow				
Radioulnar joint				
Wrist				
Metacarpophalangeal and metatarsophalangeal joints — hand and foot				
Proximal interphalangeal joints — hand and foot				
Distal interphalangeal joints — hand and foot				
Spine				
Hip				
Knee				
Ankle				

The shoulder girdle

2

Objectives

• **To identify on the skeleton important bone features of the shoulder girdle.**

• **To label on a skeletal chart the important bone features of the shoulder girdle.**

• **To draw on a skeletal chart the muscles of the shoulder girdle.**

• **To draw and indicate on a skeletal chart, using arrows, the movements of the shoulder girdle.**

• **To demonstrate, using a human subject, all of the movements of the shoulder girdle.**

• **To palpate the muscles of the shoulder girdle on a human subject.**

• **To palpate the joints of the shoulder girdle on a human subject during each movement through the full range of motion.**

Brief descriptions of the most important bones in the shoulder region will help you understand the skeletal structure and its relationship to the muscular system.

Bones FIGS. 2-1 and 2-2

Two bones are primarily involved in movements of the shoulder girdle. They are the scapula and clavicle, which generally move as a unit.

Joints FIGS. 2-1 and 2-2

When analyzing shoulder girdle (scapulothoracic) movements, it is important to realize that the scapula moves on the rib cage because the joint motion actually occurs at the sternoclavicular joint and to a lesser amount at the acromioclavicular joint.

Sternoclavicular (SC): classified as a (triaxial) arthrodial joint. It moves anteriorly 15 degrees with protraction and posteriorly 15 degrees with retraction. It moves superiorly 45 degrees with elevation and inferiorly 5 degrees with depression.

Acromioclavicular (AC): classified as an arthrodial joint. It has a 20- to 30-degree total gliding and rotational motion accompanying other shoulder girdle and shoulder joint motions.

Scapulothoracic: not a true synovial joint in that it does not have regular synovial features and its movement is totally dependent on the sternoclavicular and acromioclavicular joints. Even though scapula movement occurs as a result of motion at the SC and AC joints, the scapula can be described as having a total range of 25-degree abduction-adduction movement, 60-degree upward-downward rotation, and 55-degree elevation-depression.

FIG. 2-1 • Right shoulder girdle, anterior view.

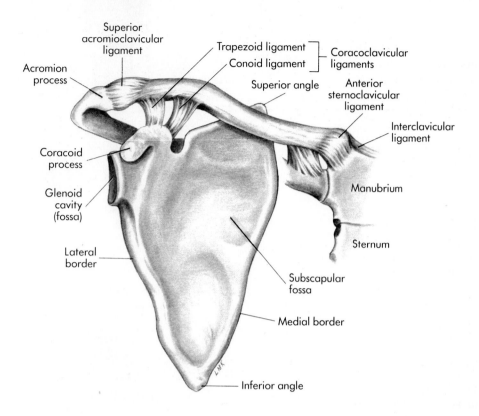

Superior
acromioclavicular
ligament

Trapezoid ligament
Conoid ligament

Coracoclavicular
ligaments

Acromion
process

Superior angle

Anterior
sternoclavicular
ligament

Interclavicular
ligament

Coracoid
process

Manubrium

Glenoid
cavity
(fossa)

Sternum

Lateral
border

Subscapular
fossa

Medial border

Inferior angle

FIG. 2-2 • Right scapula, posterior view.

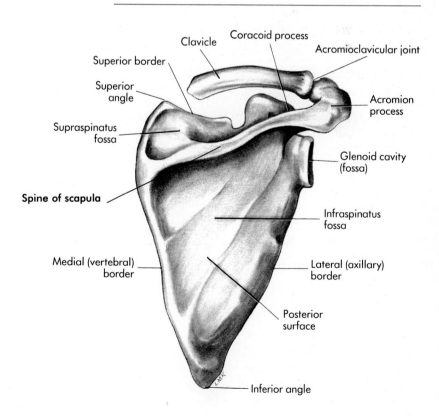

Clavicle

Coracoid process

Acromioclavicular joint

Superior border

Superior
angle

Acromion
process

Supraspinatus
fossa

Glenoid cavity
(fossa)

Spine of scapula

Infraspinatus
fossa

Medial (vertebral)
border

Lateral (axillary)
border

Posterior
surface

Inferior angle

Movements FIG. 2-3

In analyzing shoulder girdle movements, it is often helpful to focus on a specific bony landmark such as the inferior angle (posteriorly), the glenoid fossa (laterally), and the acromion process (anteriorly). All of these movements have their pivotal point where the clavicle joins the sternum at the sternoclavicular joint.

Movements of the shoulder girdle can be described as movements of the scapula.

Abduction (protraction): movement of the scapula laterally away from the spinal column.

Adduction (retraction): movement of the scapula medially toward the spinal column.

Downward rotation: returning the inferior angle medially and inferiorly toward the spinal column and the glenoid fossa to its normal position.

Upward rotation: turning the glenoid fossa upward and moving the inferior angle superiorly and laterally away from the spinal column.

Depression: downward or inferior movement, as in returning to normal position.

Elevation: upward or superior movement, as in shrugging the shoulders.

The shoulder joint and shoulder girdle work together in carrying out upper extremity activities. Table 2-1 lists the shoulder girdle movements that usually accompany shoulder joint movements.

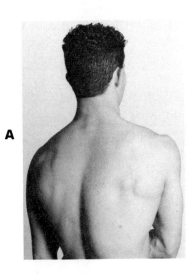

A

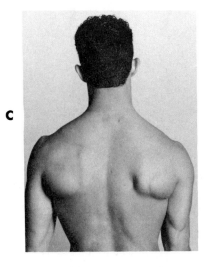

C

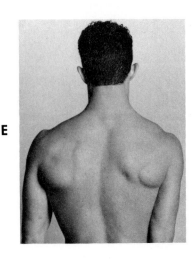

E

FIG. 2-3 • Movements of the shoulder girdle. **A,** Abduction; **B,** adduction; **C,** depression; **D,** elevation; **E,** downward rotation; **F,** upward rotation.

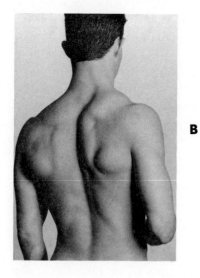

B

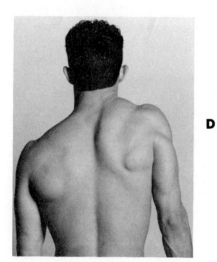

D

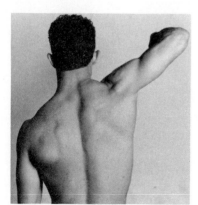

F

TABLE 2-1 • Pairing of shoulder girdle and shoulder joint movements

Shoulder joint	Shoulder girdle
Abduction	Upward rotation
Adduction	Downward rotation
Flexion	Elevation/upward rotation
Extension	Depression/downward rotation
Internal rotation	Abduction (protraction)
External rotation	Adduction (retraction)
Horizontal abduction	Adduction (retraction)
Horizontal adduction	Abduction (protraction)

Muscles

There are five muscles primarily involved in shoulder girdle movements. To avoid confusion, it is helpful to group muscles of the shoulder girdle separately from the shoulder joint. All five shoulder girdle muscles have their origin on the axial skeleton, with their insertion located on the scapula and/or the clavicle. Shoulder girdle muscles do not attach to the humerus nor do they cause actions of the shoulder joint.

The shoulder girdle muscles are essential in providing dynamic stability of the scapula so that it can serve as a relative base of support for shoulder joint activities such as throwing, batting, and blocking.

Trapezius muscle

(tra-pe'zi-us)

Origin

Upper fibers: base of skull, occipital protuberance, and posterior ligaments of neck.

Middle fibers: spinous processes of seventh cervical and upper three thoracic vertebrae.

Lower fibers: spinous processes of fourth through twelfth thoracic vertebrae.

Insertion

Upper fibers: posterior aspect of the lateral third of the clavicle.

Middle fibers: medial border of the acromion process and upper border of the scapular spine.

Lower fibers: triangular space at the base of the scapular spine.

Action

Upper fibers: elevation of the scapula.

Middle fibers: elevation, upward rotation, and adduction of the scapula.

Lower fibers: depression, adduction, and upward rotation of the scapula.

Palpation

Large area up and down from the neck region to the twelfth thoracic spine and laterally from the vertebral column to the scapula.

Innervation

Accessory nerve (cranial nerve XI) and branches of C3-4.

Functional application and strengthening

The upper fibers are a thin and relatively weak part of the muscle. They provide some elevation of the clavicle. As a mover of the head, they are of minor importance.

The middle fibers are stronger and thicker and provide strong elevation, upward rotation, and adduction (retraction) of the scapula.

The lower fibers assist in adduction (retraction) and rotate the scapula upward.

When all the parts of the trapezius are working together, they tend to pull upward and adduct at the same time. Typical action of the trapezius muscle is fixation of the scapula for deltoid action. Continuous action in upward rotation of the scapula permits the arms to be raised over the head. The muscle is always used in preventing the glenoid fossae from being pulled down during the lifting of objects with the arms. It is also typically seen in action during the holding of an object overhead. Holding the arm at the side horizontally shows typical fixation of the scapula by the trapezius muscle, while the deltoid muscle holds the arm in that position. The muscle is used strenuously when lifting with the hands, as in picking up a heavy wheelbarrow. The trapezius must prevent the scapula from being pulled downward. Carrying objects on the tip of the shoulder also calls this muscle into play. Strengthening of the upper and middle fibers can be accomplished through shoulder-shrugging exercises. The middle and lower fibers can be strengthened through bent rowing from a prone or semiprone position and side arm shoulder joint abduction exercises.

FIG. 2-4 • Trapezius muscle. *O,* Origin; *I,* insertion.

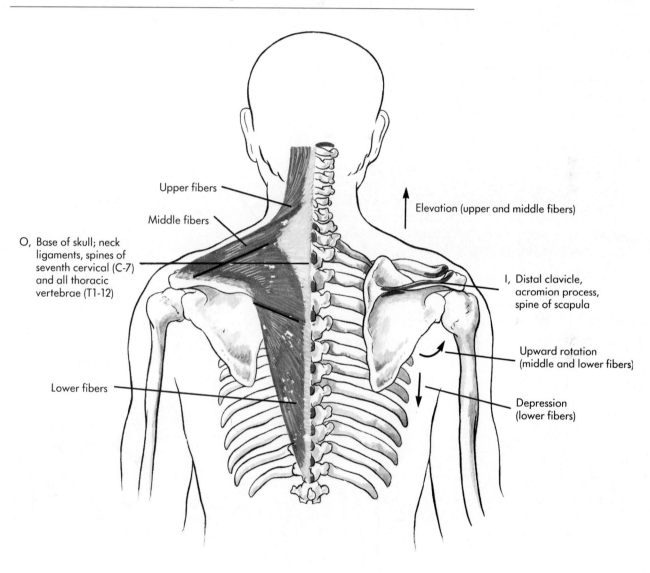

Upper fibers

Middle fibers

O, Base of skull; neck
ligaments, spines of
seventh cervical (C-7)
and all thoracic
vertebrae (T1-12)

Lower fibers

Elevation (upper and middle fibers)

I, Distal clavicle,
acromion process,
spine of scapula

Upward rotation
(middle and lower fibers)

Depression
(lower fibers)

Levator scapulae muscle FIG. 2-5

(le-va'tor scap'u-lae)

Origin

Transverse processes of the upper four cervical vertebrae.

Insertion

Medial border of the scapula above the base of the scapular spine.

Action

Elevates the medial margin of the scapula.

Palpation

Cannot be palpated; under the trapezius muscle.

Innervation

Dorsal scapula nerve C5 and branches of C3 and C4.

Functional application and strengthening

Shrugging the shoulders calls the levator scapulae muscle into play, along with the upper trapezius muscle. Fixation of the scapula by the pectoralis minor muscle allows the levator scapulae muscles on both sides to extend the neck or to flex laterally if used on one side only.

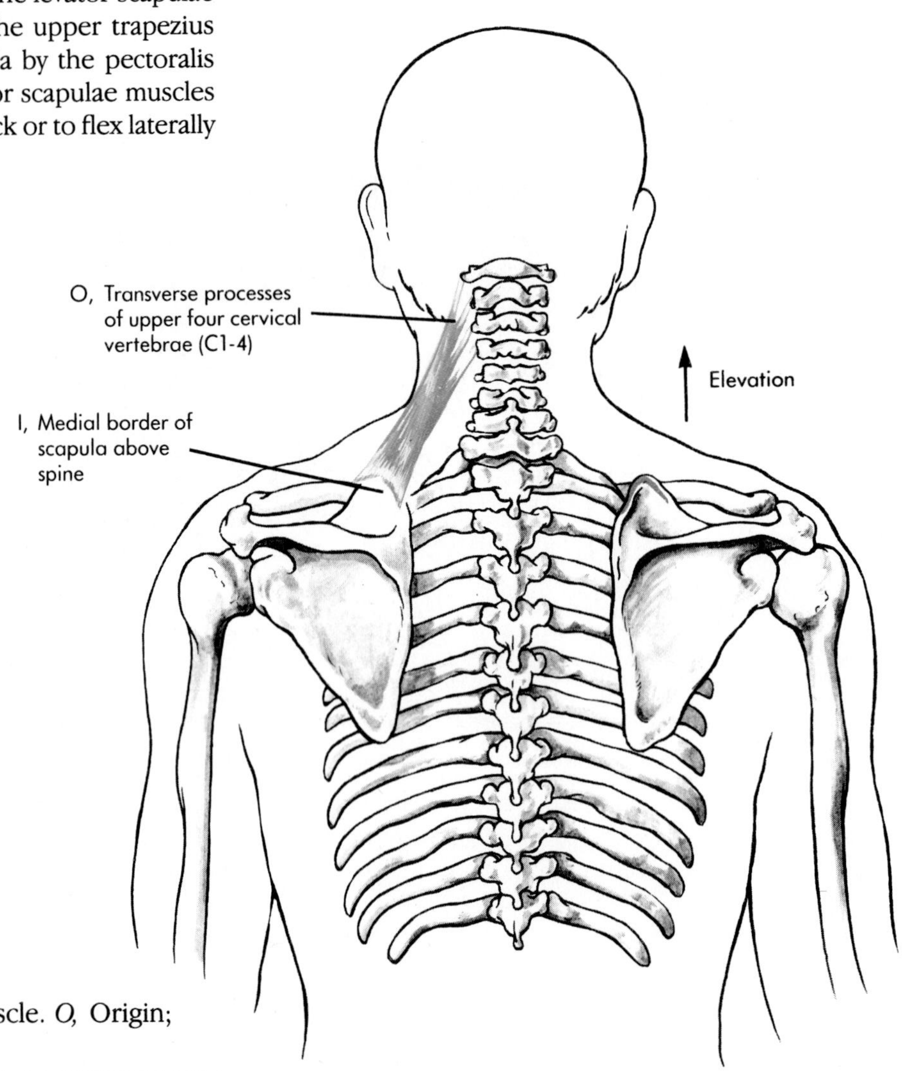

O, Transverse processes of upper four cervical vertebrae (C1-4)

Elevation

I, Medial border of scapula above spine

FIG. 2-5 • Levator scapulae muscle. *O*, Origin; *I*, insertion.

Rhomboid muscles—major and minor FIG. 2-6

(rom'boyd)

Origin

Spinous processes of the last cervical and the first five thoracic vertebrae.

Insertion

Medial border of the scapula, below the spine.

Action

The rhomboid major and minor muscles work together.

Adduction (retraction): draw the scapula toward the spinal column; elevate slightly as they adduct.

Rotation downward: from the upward rotated position; they draw the scapula in a downward rotation.

Palpation

Cannot be palpated; under the trapezius muscle.

Innervation

Dorsal scapula nerve (C5).

Functional application and strengthening

The rhomboid muscles fix the scapula in adduction (retraction) when the muscles of the shoulder joint adduct or extend the arm. These muscles are used powerfully in chinning. As one hangs from the horizontal bar, suspended by the hands, the scapula tends to be pulled away from the top of the chest. When the chinning movement begins, it is the rhomboid muscles that draw the medial border of the scapula down and back toward the spinal column. Note their favorable position to do this.

The trapezius and rhomboid muscles working together produce adduction with slight elevation of the scapula. To prevent this elevation, the latissimus dorsi muscle is called into play.

Chin-ups and dips are excellent exercises for developing this muscle.

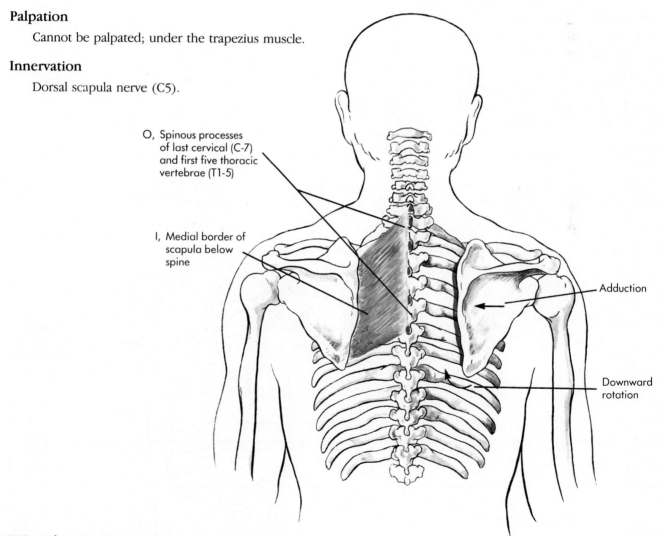

O, Spinous processes of last cervical (C-7) and first five thoracic vertebrae (T1-5)

I, Medial border of scapula below spine

Adduction

Downward rotation

FIG. 2-6 • Rhomboid muscles (major and minor). *O,* Origin; *I,* insertion.

Serratus anterior muscle FIG. 2-7

(ser-a′tus an-tir′e-or)

Origin

Surface of the upper nine ribs at the side of the chest.

Insertion

Anterior aspect of the whole length of the medial border of the scapula.

Action

Abduction (protraction): draws the medial border of the scapula away from the vertebrae.

Rotation upward: longer, lower fibers tend to draw the inferior angle of the scapula farther away from the vertebrae, thus rotating the scapula upward slightly.

Palpation

Front and lateral side of the chest below the fifth and sixth ribs.

Innervation

Long thoracic nerve (C5,6,7).

Functional application and strengthening

The serratus anterior muscle is used commonly in movements drawing the scapula forward with slight upward rotation, such as throwing a baseball, shooting and guarding in basketball, and tackling in football. It works along with the pectoralis major muscle in typical action, such as throwing a baseball.

The serratus anterior muscle is used strongly in doing push-ups, especially in the last 5 to 10 degrees of motion. The bench press and overhead press are good exercises for this muscle. A winged scapula condition indicates a definite weakness of the serratus anterior.

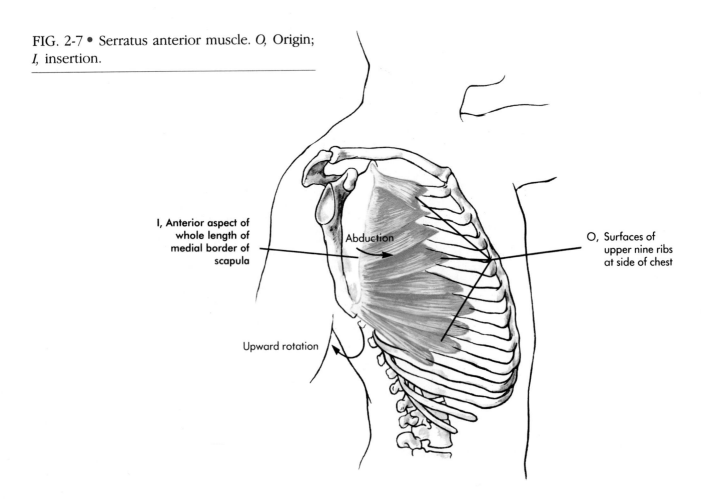

FIG. 2-7 • Serratus anterior muscle. *O,* Origin; *I,* insertion.

I, Anterior aspect of whole length of medial border of scapula

Abduction

O, Surfaces of upper nine ribs at side of chest

Upward rotation

Pectoralis minor muscle

(pek-to-ra′lis mi′nor)

Origin

Anterior surfaces of the third to fifth ribs.

Insertion

Coracoid process of the scapula.

Action

Abduction (protraction): draws the scapula forward and tends to tilt the lower border away from the ribs.

Downward rotation: as it abducts, it draws the scapula downward.

Depression: when the scapula is rotated upward, it assists in depression.

Palpation

Difficult to palpate, but can be palpated under the pectoralis major muscle in the pit of the shoulder during powerful downward movement.

Innervation

Medial pectoral nerve (C8-T1).

Functional application and strengthening

The pectoralis minor muscle is used, along with the serratus anterior muscle, in true abduction (protraction) without rotation. This is seen particularly in movements such as push-ups. True abduction of the scapula is necessary. Therefore the serratus anterior draws the scapula forward with a tendency toward upward rotation, the pectoralis minor pulls forward with a tendency toward downward rotation, and the two pulling together give true abduction, which is necessary in push-ups. These muscles will be seen working together in most movements of pushing with the hands.

FIG. 2-8 • Pectoralis minor muscle. *O,* Origin; *I,* insertion.

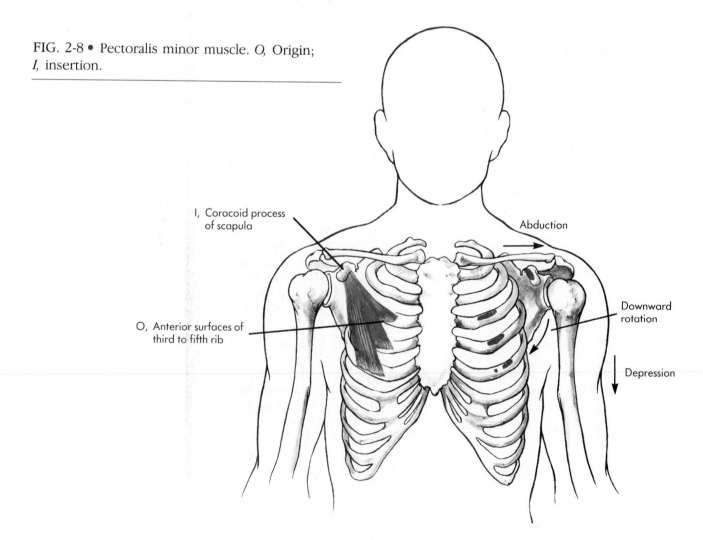

I, Coracoid process of scapula

O, Anterior surfaces of third to fifth rib

Abduction

Downward rotation

Depression

Worksheet exercises

As an aid to learning, for in-class or out-of-class assignments, or for testing, tearout worksheets are found at the end of the text (pp. 215 and 216).

Skeletal worksheet (no. 1)

Draw and label on the worksheet the following listed muscles:
a. Trapezius
b. Rhomboid major and minor
c. Serratus anterior
d. Levator scapulae
e. Pectoralis minor

Human figure worksheet (no. 2)

Label the circles next to the arrows with the appropriate letter that corresponds to the movements of the shoulder girdle indicated by the arrow:
a. Adduction (retraction)
b. Abduction (protraction)
c. Rotation upward
d. Rotation downward
e. Elevation
f. Depression

Laboratory and review exercises

1. Locate the following prominent skeletal features on a human skeleton and on a subject:
   a. **Scapula**
      (1) Medial border
      (2) Inferior angle
      (3) Superior angle
      (4) Coracoid process
      (5) Spine of scapula
      (6) Glenoid cavity
      (7) Acromion process
      (8) Supraspinatus fossa
      (9) Infraspinatus fossa
   b. **Clavicle**
      (1) Sternal end
      (2) Acromial end
   c. **Joints**
      (1) Sternoclavicular joint
      (2) Acromioclavicular joint
2. How and where do you palpate the following muscles on a human subject?
   a. Serratus anterior
   b. Trapezius
   c. Rhomboid major and minor
   d. Levator scapulae
   e. Pectoralis minor
      NOTE: *How* means resisting a primary movement of the muscle. Some muscles have several primary movements, such as the trapezius rotation upward and adduction. *Where* refers to the location on the body where the muscle can be felt.
3. Palpate the sternoclavicular and acromioclavicular joint movements and the muscles primarily involved while demonstrating the following shoulder girdle movements:
   a. Adduction
   b. Abduction
   c. Rotation upward
   d. Rotation downward
   e. Elevation
   f. Depression
4. List the muscles that are primarily responsible for the following actions:
   a. Shoulder girdle adduction
   b. Shoulder girdle abduction
   c. Shoulder girdle elevation
   d. Shoulder girdle depression
   e. Shoulder girdle upward rotation
   f. Shoulder girdle downward rotation
5. Fill in the movements and muscle actions of the shoulder girdle on the chart at the right. List the muscles primarily involved in each movement.

Muscle analysis chart • Shoulder girdle

Shoulder girdle
Abduction
Adduction
Elevation
Depression
Upward rotation
Downward rotation

References

Daniels L, Worthingham C: Muscle testing techniques of manual examination, ed 5, 1989, Philadelphia, Saunders.

Lehmkuhl LD, Smith LK: Brunnstrom's clinical kinesiology, ed 4, Philadelphia, 1983, Davis.

McMurtrie H, Rikel JK: The coloring review guide to human anatomy, 1991, Dubuque, Ia, Brown.

Norkin CC, Levangie PK: Joint structure and function—a comprehensive analysis, Philadelphia, 1983, Davis.

Rasch PJ: Kinesiology and applied anatomy, ed 7, 1989, Philadelphia, Lea & Febiger.

Soderburg GL: Kinesiology—application to pathological motion, Baltimore, 1986, Williams & Wilkins.

The shoulder joint

Objectives

- To identify on a human skeleton or human subject the most important bone structures of the shoulder joint.

- To label on a skeletal chart the important bone structures of the shoulder joint.

- To draw and label on a skeletal chart the muscles of the shoulder joint.

- To demonstrate with a fellow student all of the movements of the shoulder joints.

- To label a human skeletal chart with arrows to indicate the movements of the shoulder joint.

- To organize and list the muscles that produce the movements of the shoulder girdle and the shoulder joint.

The only attachment of the shoulder joint to the axial skeleton is with the clavicle at the sternoclavicular joint. Movements of the shoulder joint are many and varied. It is unusual to have movement of the humerus without scapula movement. When the humerus is flexed and abducted, the scapula is elevated, rotated upward, and abducted. Adduction and extension of the humerus results in depression, rotation downward, and adduction of the scapula. The scapula abducts with humeral internal rotation and horizontal adduction. Scapula adduction accompanies exter-

nal rotation and horizontal abduction of the humerus. Refer to Table 2-1.

Because the shoulder joint has such a wide range of motion in so many different planes, it also has a significant amount of laxity, which often results in instability problems such as rotator cuff impingement, subluxations, or dislocations. The price of mobility is stability. The concept that the more mobile a joint is, the less stable it is and that the more stable it is, the less mobile it is applies generally throughout the body but particularly in the shoulder joint.

Bones FIGS. 2-1 and 3-1

The scapula, clavicle, and humerus serve as attachments for most of the muscles of the shoulder joint.

Joints FIG. 3-1

The shoulder joint, specifically known as the glenohumeral joint, is a multiaxial ball-and-socket joint classified as enarthrodial. Its stability is enhanced slightly by the glenoid labrum, a cartilagenous ring that surrounds the glenoid fossa just inside its periphery. It is further stabilized by the glenohumeral ligaments, especially anteriorly and inferiorly.

Movement of the humerus from the side position is common in throwing, tackling, and striking activities. Flexion and extension of the shoulder joint are performed frequently when supporting the body weight in a hanging position or in a movement from a prone position on the ground.

Determining the exact range of each movement for the glenohumeral joint is difficult because of the accompanying shoulder girdle movement. However, the glenohumeral joint movements are generally thought to be in the following ranges: 90 to 95 degrees abduction, 0 degree adduction (prevented by the trunk) or 75 degrees anterior to the trunk, 40 to 60 degrees of extension, 90 to 100 degrees of flexion, 70 to 90 degrees of internal and external rotation, 45 degrees of horizontal abduction, and 135 degrees of horizontal adduction.

The shoulder joint is frequently injured because of its anatomical design. A number of factors contribute to its injury rate, including the shallowness of the glenoid fossa, the laxity of the ligamentous structures (which is necessary to accommodate its wide range of motion), and the lack of strength and endurance in the muscles, which are essential in providing dynamic stability to the joint.

A frequent injury is to the rotator cuff. The subscapularis, supraspinatus, infraspinatus, and teres minor muscles make up the rotator cuff. They are small muscles that attach to the front, top, and rear of the head of the humerus. Their point of insertion makes them able to rotate the humerus, an essential movement in this freely movable joint.

FIG. 3-1 • Right glenohumeral joint, anterior view.

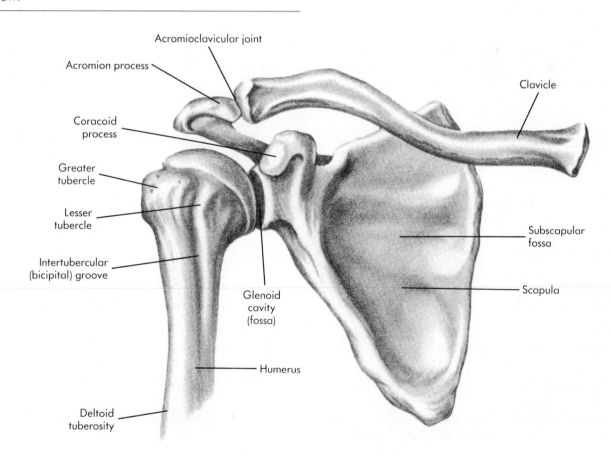

Acromioclavicular joint

Acromion process

Coracoid process

Clavicle

Greater tubercle

Lesser tubercle

Intertubercular (bicipital) groove

Subscapular fossa

Glenoid cavity (fossa)

Scapula

Humerus

Deltoid tuberosity

Movements

Abduction: upward lateral movement of the humerus out to the side away from the body.

Adduction: downward movement of the humerus medially toward the body from abduction.

Flexion: movement of the humerus straight anteriorly.

Extension: movement of the humerus straight posteriorly.

Horizontal adduction (flexion): movement of the humerus in a horizontal or transverse plane toward and across the chest.

Horizontal abduction (extension): movement of the humerus in a horizontal or transverse plane away from the chest.

External rotation: movement of the humerus laterally around its long axis away from the midline.

Internal rotation: movement of the humerus medially around its long axis toward the midline.

FIG. 3-2 • Movements of the shoulder joint. **A**, Flexion; **B**, extension; **C**, adduction; **D**, abduction; **E**, internal rotation; **F**, external rotation; **G**, horizontal adduction; **H**, horizontal abduction.

A
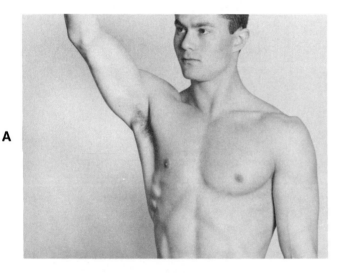

B
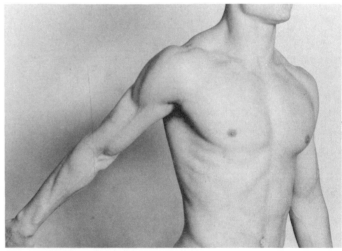

C
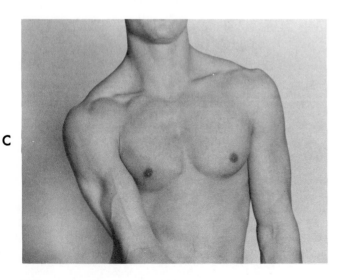

D
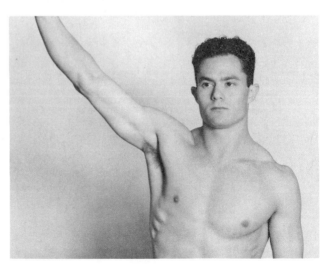

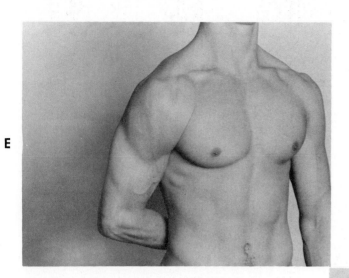

E

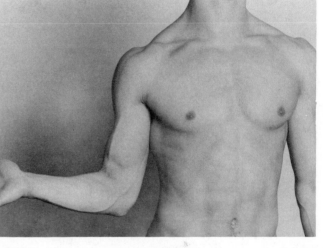

F

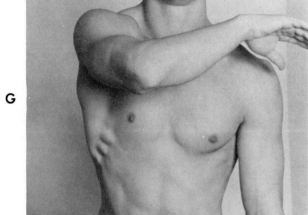

G

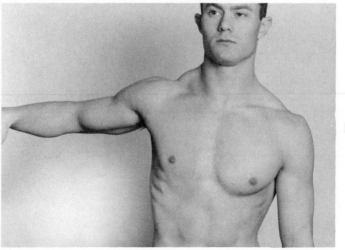

H

Muscles

When attempting to learn and understand the muscles of the glenohumeral joint, it may be helpful to group them according to their location and function. All of the muscles that originate on the scapula and clavicle may be thought of as intrinsic glenohumeral muscles. The intrinsic muscles include the deltoid, the coracobrachialis, the teres major, and the rotator cuff group, which is composed of the subscapularis, the supraspinatus, the infraspinatus, and the teres minor.

Muscle identification

In Figs. 3-3 and 3-5, identify the anterior and posterior muscles of the shoulder joint and shoulder girdle. Compare Fig. 3-3 with Fig. 3-4 and Fig. 3-5 with Fig. 3-6.

FIG. 3-3 • Anterior shoulder joint and shoulder girdle muscles.

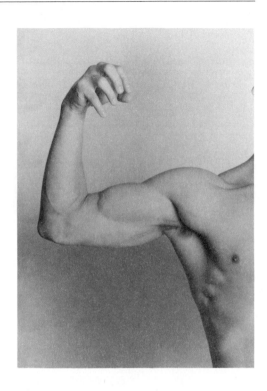

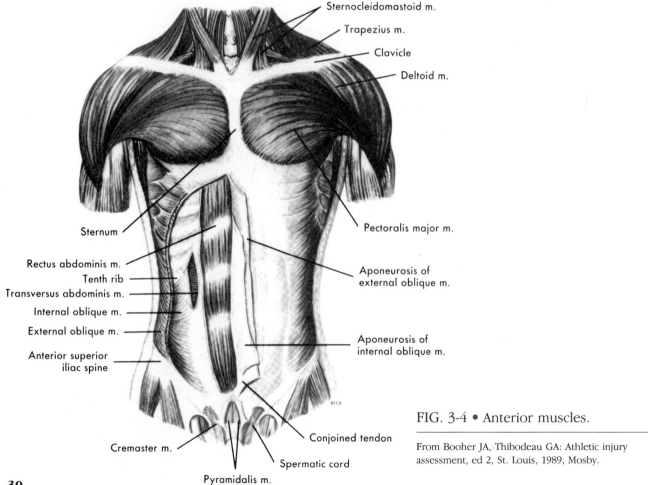

- Sternocleidomastoid m.
- Trapezius m.
- Clavicle
- Deltoid m.
- Pectoralis major m.
- Sternum
- Rectus abdominis m.
- Tenth rib
- Transversus abdominis m.
- Internal oblique m.
- External oblique m.
- Anterior superior iliac spine
- Aponeurosis of external oblique m.
- Aponeurosis of internal oblique m.
- Cremaster m.
- Conjoined tendon
- Spermatic cord
- Pyramidalis m.

FIG. 3-4 • Anterior muscles.

From Booher JA, Thibodeau GA: Athletic injury assessment, ed 2, St. Louis, 1989, Mosby.

FIG. 3-5 • Posterior shoulder joint and shoulder girdle muscles.

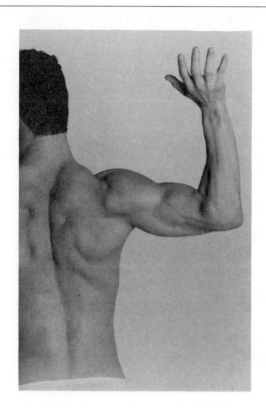

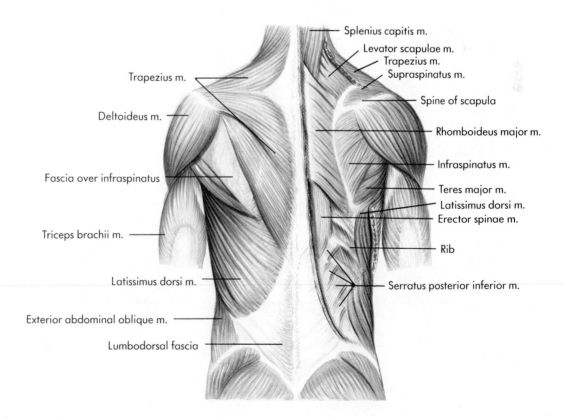

FIG. 3-6 • Posterior muscles.

Splenius capitis m.
Levator scapulae m.
Trapezius m.
Supraspinatus m.
Spine of scapula
Rhomboideus major m.
Infraspinatus m.
Teres major m.
Latissimus dorsi m.
Erector spinae m.
Rib
Serratus posterior inferior m.

Trapezius m.
Deltoideus m.
Fascia over infraspinatus
Triceps brachii m.
Latissimus dorsi m.
Exterior abdominal oblique m.
Lumbodorsal fascia

Deltoid muscle FIG. 3-7

(del-toyd')

Origin

Anterior lateral third of the clavicle, lateral aspect of the acromion, and inferior edge of the spine of the scapula.

Insertion

Deltoid tuberosity on the lateral humerus.

Action

Abduction: entire muscle moves arm laterally away from the body.

Flexion: anterior fibers move the arm straight anteriorly.

Horizontal adduction: anterior fibers move the arm in a horizontal plane toward the chest.

Internal rotation: anterior fibers assist in rotating the arm toward the chest.

Extension: posterior fibers move the arm straight posteriorly.

Horizontal abduction: posterior fibers move the arm in a horizontal plane away from the chest.

External rotation: posterior fibers assist in rotating the arm away from the chest.

Palpation

Over the head of the humerus from the anterior to the posterior side.

Innervation

Axillary nerve (C5,6).

Functional application and strengthening

The deltoid muscle is used commonly in any lifting movement. The trapezius muscle stabilizes the scapula as the deltoid pulls on the humerus. The anterior fibers of the deltoid muscle flex and internally rotate the humerus. The posterior fibers extend and externally rotate the humerus. The anterior fibers also horizontally adduct the humerus while the posterior fibers horizontally abduct it.

This muscle is used in all lifting movements if the arms are at the side in lifting.

Any movement of the humerus on the scapula will involve part or all of the deltoid muscle.

Lifting the humerus from the side to the position of abduction is a typical action of the deltoid. Side-arm dumbell raises are excellent for strengthening the deltoid, especially the middle fibers. By abducting the arm in a slightly horizontally adducted (30 degrees) position, the anterior deltoid fibers can be emphasized. The posterior fibers can be strengthened better by abducting the arm in a slightly horizontally abducted (30 degrees) position.

FIG. 3-7 • Deltoid muscle. *O*, Origin; *I*, insertion.

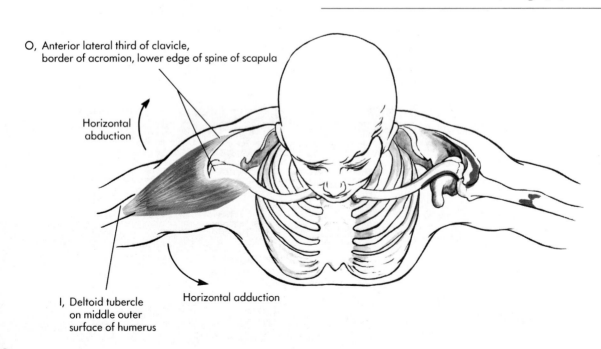

O, Anterior lateral third of clavicle, border of acromion, lower edge of spine of scapula

Horizontal abduction

I, Deltoid tubercle on middle outer surface of humerus

Horizontal adduction

Coracobrachialis muscle FIG. 3-8

(kor-a-ko-bra'ki-a'lis)

Origin

Coracoid process of the scapula.

Insertion

Middle of the medial border of the humeral shaft.

Action

Flexion: moves the arm straight anteriorly.
Adduction: assists in pulling the arm medially toward the body.
Horizontal adduction: moves the arm horizontally across the chest.

Palpation

Difficult to palpate.

Innervation

Musculotaneous nerve (C5,6,7).

Functional application and strengthening

The coracobrachialis is not a powerful muscle, but it does assist in flexion and adduction and is most functional in moving the arm horizontally toward and across the chest. It is best strengthened by horizontally adducting the arm against resistance such as in bench pressing. It may also be strengthened by performing lat pulls.

FIG. 3-8 • Coracobrachialis muscle. *O*, Origin; *I*, insertion.

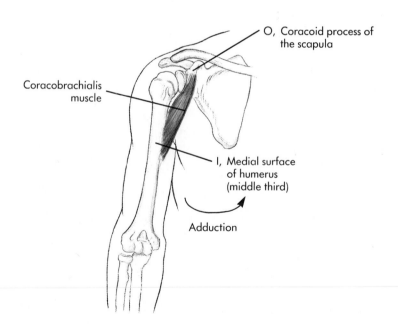

O, Coracoid process of the scapula

Coracobrachialis muscle

I, Medial surface of humerus (middle third)

Adduction

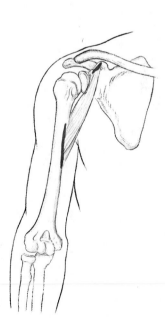

Supraspinatus muscle FIG. 3-9

(su'pra-spi-na'tus)

Origin

Medial two thirds of the supraspinatus fossa.

Insertion

Superiorly on the greater tubercle of the humerus.

Action

Weak abduction and stabilization of the humeral head in the glenoid fossa.

Palpation

Cannot be palpated; under the deltoid muscle distally and under the trapezius proximally.

Innervation

Suprascapula nerve (C5).

Functional application and strengthening

The supraspinatus muscle holds the head of the humerus in the glenoid fossa. In throwing movements it provides important dynamic stability by maintaining the proper relationship between the humeral head and the glenoid fossa. In the cocking phase of throwing, there is a tendency for the humeral head to sublux anteriorly. In the follow-through phase, the humeral head tends to move posteriorly.

The supraspinatus, along with the other rotator cuff muscles, must have excellent strength and endurance to prevent abnormal and excessive movement of the humeral head in the fossa.

The supraspinatus is the most often injured rotator cuff muscle. Acute severe injuries may occur with trauma to the shoulder. However, mild-to-moderate strains or tears often occur with athletic activity, particularly if the activity involves repetitious overhead movements such as throwing or swimming.

Injury or weakness in the supraspinatus may be detected when the athlete attempts to substitute the scapula elevators and upward rotators to obtain humeral abduction. Inability to smoothly abduct the arm against resistance is indicative of possible rotator cuff injury.

The supraspinatus muscle may be called into play whenever the middle fibers of the deltoid muscle are used. An "empty-can exercise" may be used to emphasize supraspinatus action. This is performed by internally rotating the humerus, followed by abducting the arm to 90 degrees in a 30- to 45-degree horizontally adducted position as if one were emptying a can.

FIG. 3-9 • Supraspinatus muscle. *O,* Origin; *I,* insertion.

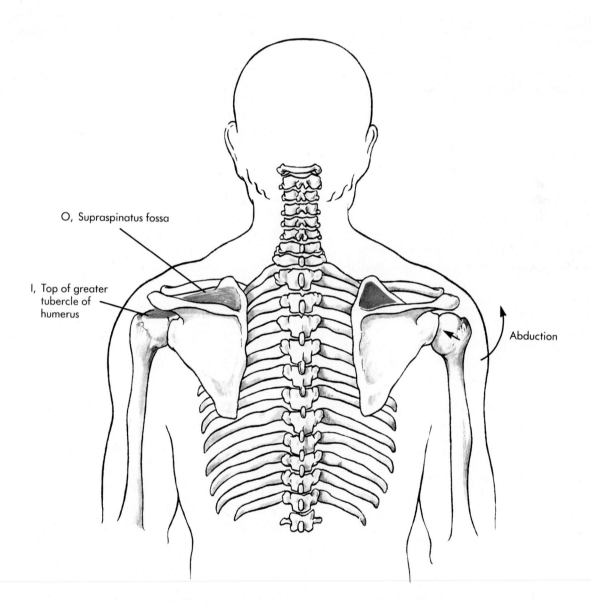

O, Supraspinatus fossa

I, Top of greater tubercle of humerus

Abduction

Infraspinatus muscle FIG. 3-10

(in'fra-spi-na'tus)

Origin

Medial aspect of the infraspinatus fossa just below the spine of the scapula.

Insertion

Posteriorly on the greater tubercle of the humerus.

Action

External rotation: rotates the humerus laterally.
Horizontal abduction: moves the humerus in a horizontal plane away from the chest.
Extension: moves the humerus posteriorly from the flexed or neutral position.

Palpation

Immediately below the spine of the scapula and the posterior fibers of the deltoid muscle.

Innervation

Suprascapula nerve (C5,6).

Functional application and strengthening

The infraspinatus and teres minor muscles are effective when the rhomboid muscles stabilize the scapula. When the humerus is rotated outward, the rhomboid muscles flatten the scapula to the back and fixate it so that the humerus may be rotated.

The infraspinatus is vital to maintaining the posterior stability of the glenohumeral joint. It is the most powerful of the external rotators and is the second most commonly injured rotator cuff muscle.

Exercises in which the arms are pulled down bring the infraspinatus, teres major, and latissimus dorsi into powerful contraction. Chinning, rope climbing, and dips on parallel bars are good exercises for these muscles. Both the infraspinatus and the teres minor can best be strengthened by externally rotating the arm against resistance in the 0-degree abducted position and the 90-degree abducted position.

FIG. 3-10 • Infraspinatus muscle. *O*, Origin; *I*, insertion.

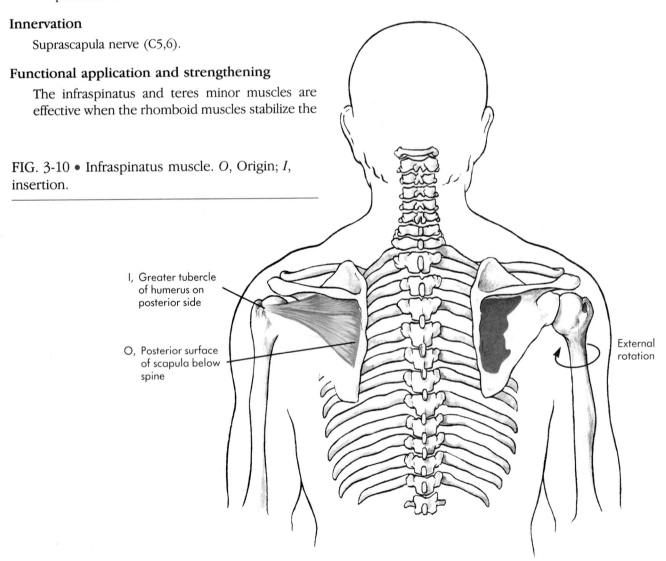

I, Greater tubercle of humerus on posterior side

O, Posterior surface of scapula below spine

External rotation

Teres minor muscle FIG. 3-11

(te'rez mi'nor)

Origin

Posteriorly on the upper and middle aspect of the lateral border of the scapula.

Insertion

Posteriorly on the greater tubercle of the humerus.

Action

External rotation: rotates the humerus laterally.

Horizontal abduction: moves the humerus in a horizontal plane away from the chest.

Extension: moves the humerus posteriorly from the flexed or neutral position.

Palpation

Between the posterior deltoid and the lateral scapula border.

Innervation

Axillary nerve (C5,6).

Functional application and strengthening

The teres minor functions very similarly to the infraspinatus in providing dynamic posterior stability to the glenohumeral joint. Both of these muscles perform the same actions together. The teres minor is strengthened with the same exercises that are used in strengthening the infraspinatus.

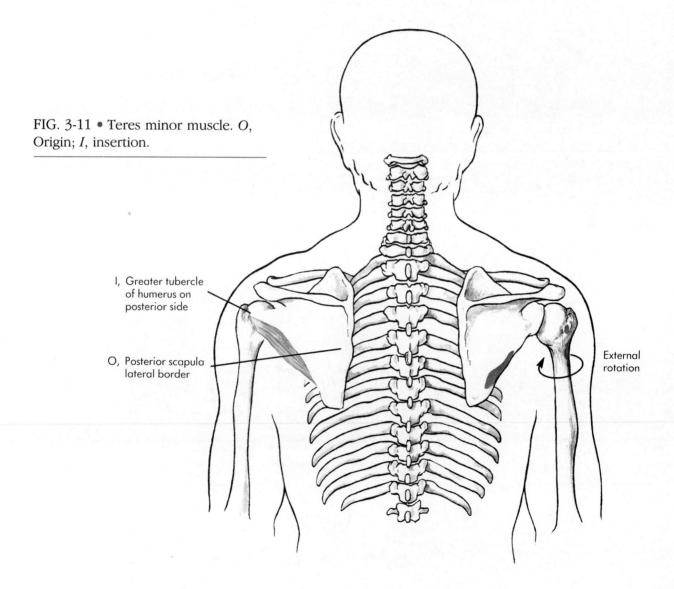

FIG. 3-11 • Teres minor muscle. *O*, Origin; *I*, insertion.

I, Greater tubercle of humerus on posterior side

O, Posterior scapula lateral border

External rotation

Subscapularis muscle

(sub-skap-u-la′ris)

Origin

Entire anterior surface of the subscapular fossa.

Insertion

Lesser tubercle of the humerus.

Action

Internal rotation: rotates the humerus medially.
Adduction: draws the arm down toward the body
from the abducted position.
Extension: assists in moving the humerus posteriorly
from the flexed position.

Palpation

Cannot be palpated.

Innervation

Upper and lower subscapular nerve (C5,6).

Functional application and strengthening

The subscapularis muscle, another rotator cuff muscle, holds the head of the humerus in the glenoid fossa from in front and below. It acts with the latissimus dorsi and teres major muscles in its typical movement but is less powerful in its action because of its proximity to the joint. The muscle also requires the help of the rhomboid in stabilizing the scapula to make it effective in the described movements. It may be strengthened with exercises similar to those used for the latissimus dorsi and teres major such as rope climbing and lat pulls. A specific exercise for its development is done by internally rotating the arm against resistance in the 0-degree abducted beside-the-body position.

FIG. 3-12 • Subscapularis muscle. *O*, Origin; *I*, insertion.

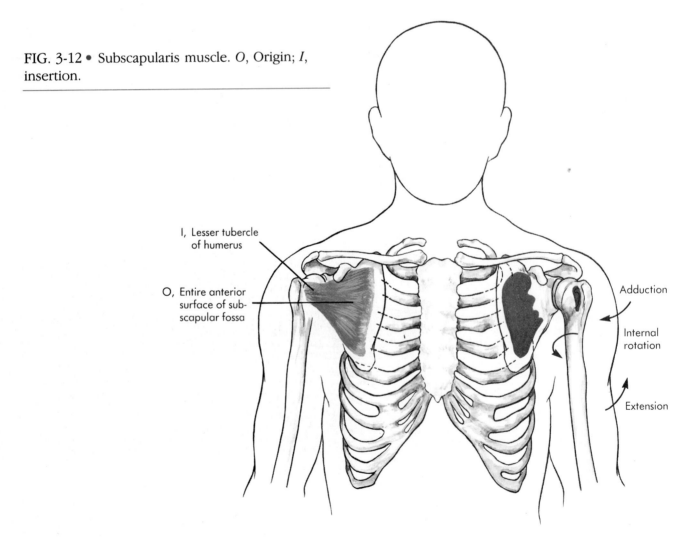

I, Lesser tubercle
of humerus

O, Entire anterior
surface of sub-
scapular fossa

Adduction

Internal
rotation

Extension

Teres major muscle FIG. 3-13

(te'rez ma'jor)

Origin

Posteriorly on the inferior third of the lateral border of the scapula and just superior to the inferior angle.

Insertion

Medial lip of the intertubercular groove of the humerus.

Action

Extension: moves the arm from the flexed position to the posteriorly extended position.

Internal rotation: rotates the humerus medially.

Adduction: draws the arm from the abducted position down to the side and toward the midline of the body.

Palpation

Posterior surface, diagonally upward from the inferior angle of the scapula.

Innervation

Lower subscapular nerve (C5,6).

Functional application and strengthening

The teres major muscle is effective only when the rhomboid muscles stabilize the scapula or move the scapula in a downward rotation. Otherwise the scapula would move forward to meet the arm.

This muscle works effectively with the latissimus dorsi. It assists the latissimus dorsi, pectoralis major, and subscapularis in adducting, internally rotating, and extending the humerus. It is said to be latissimus dorsi's "little helper." It may be strengthened by lat pulls, rope climbing, and internal rotation exercises against resistance.

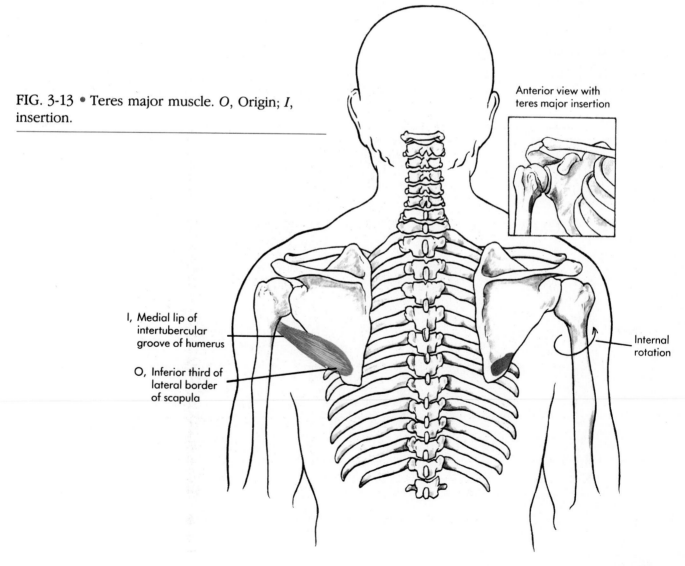

FIG. 3-13 • Teres major muscle. *O*, Origin; *I*, insertion.

Anterior view with teres major insertion

I, Medial lip of intertubercular groove of humerus

O, Inferior third of lateral border of scapula

Internal rotation

Latissimus dorsi muscle FIG. 3-14

(lat-is'i-mus dor'si)

Origin

Posterior crest of the ilium, back of the sacrum and spinous processes of the lumbar and lower six thoracic vertebrae (T6-12); slips from the lower three ribs.

Insertion

Medial side of the intertubercular groove of the humerus.

Action

Adduction: draws the arm from the abducted position down to the side and toward the midline of the body.

Extension: moves the arm from the flexed position to the posteriorly extended position.

Internal rotation: rotates the humerus medially.

Horizontal abduction: moves the arm in a horizontal plane away from the chest.

Palpation

Lateral, posterior aspect of the trunk below the armpit.

Innervation

Thoracodorsal (C6,7,8).

Functional application and strengthening

The latissimus dorsi muscle has strong action in downward rotation and adduction of the humerus. It is one of the most important extensor muscles of the humerus and contracts powerfully in chinning.

Exercises in which the arms are pulled down bring the latissimus dorsi muscle into powerful contraction. Chinning, rope climbing, dips on parallel bars, and other uprise movements on the horizontal bar are good examples. In barbell exercises, the basic rowing and pullover exercises are good for developing the "lats." Pulling an overhead pulley system bar down toward the shoulders is a common exercise for this muscle known as lat pulls.

FIG. 3-14 • Latissimus dorsi muscle. *O*, Origin; *I*, insertion.

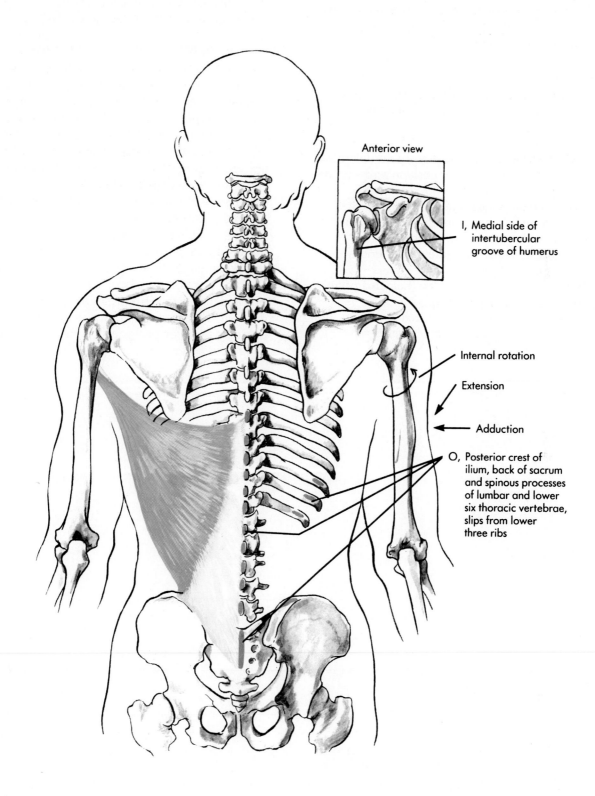

Anterior view

I, Medial side of intertubercular groove of humerus

Internal rotation

Extension

Adduction

O, Posterior crest of ilium, back of sacrum and spinous processes of lumbar and lower six thoracic vertebrae, slips from lower three ribs

Pectoralis major muscle FIG. 3-15

(pek-to-ra′lis ma′jor)

Origin

Upper fibers (clavicular head): medial half of the anterior surface of the clavicle.

Lower fibers (sternal head): anterior surface of the costal cartilages of the first six ribs, and adjoining portion of the sternum.

Insertion

Flat tendon 2 or 3 inches wide to the outer lip of the intertubercular groove of the humerus.

Action

Horizontal adduction: draws the arm powerfully from the horizontally abducted position across to the chest.

Internal rotation: rotates the humerus medially.

Adduction: moves the arm from the abducted position down toward the body.

Flexion: upper fibers move the arm anteriorly from the side.

Extension: lower fibers move the humerus posteriorly from the flexed position.

Abduction: once the arm is abducted 90 degrees, the upper fibers assist in further abduction.

Palpation

Broad area of the chest region between the clavicle and the sixth rib.

Innervation

Upper fibers: lateral pectoral nerve (C5,6,7).
Lower fibers: medial pectoral nerve (C8,T1).

Functional application and strengthening

The pectoralis major muscle aids the serratus anterior muscle in drawing the scapula forward as it moves the humerus in flexion and internal rotation. Typical action is shown in throwing a baseball. As the humerus is flexed, it is internally rotated, and the scapula is drawn forward with upward rotation. It also works as a helper of the latissimus dorsi muscle when extending and adducting the humerus from a raised position.

The pectoralis major and the anterior deltoid work closely together. The pectoralis major is used powerfully in push-ups, pull-ups, throwing, and serving in tennis. With a barbell, the subject takes a supine position on a bench with the arm at the side and moves the arm to a horizontally adducted position. This exercise, known as bench pressing, is widely used for pectoralis major development.

FIG. 3-15 • Pectoralis major muscle. *O*, Origin; *I*, insertion.

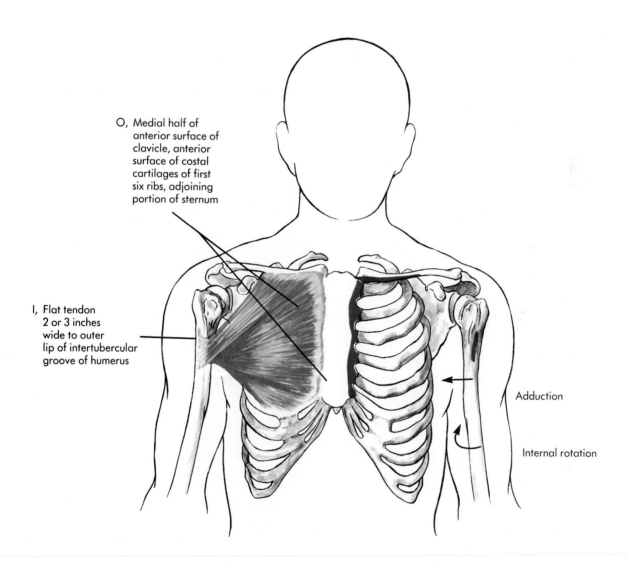

O, Medial half of anterior surface of clavicle, anterior surface of costal cartilages of first six ribs, adjoining portion of sternum

I, Flat tendon 2 or 3 inches wide to outer lip of intertubercular groove of humerus

Adduction

Internal rotation

Worksheet exercises

As an aid to learning, for in-class or out-of-class assignments, or for testing, tearout worksheets are found at the end of the text (pp. 217 and 218).

Skeletal worksheet (no. 1)

Draw and label on the worksheet the following muscles:
a. Deltoid
b. Supraspinatus
c. Subscapularis
d. Teres major
e. Infraspinatus
f. Teres minor
g. Latissimus dorsi
h. Pectoralis major
i. Coracobrachialis

Human figure worksheet (no. 2)

Label and indicate by arrows the following listed movements of the shoulder joint:
a. Abduction
b. Adduction
c. Flexion
d. Extension
e. Horizontal adduction
f. Horizontal abduction
g. Internal rotation
h. External rotation

Laboratory and review exercises

1. Locate the following parts of the humerus and scapula on a human skeleton and on a subject:
   a. **Skeleton**
      (1) Greater tubercle
      (2) Lesser tubercle
      (3) Neck
      (4) Shaft
      (5) Intertubercular groove
      (6) Medial epicondyle
      (7) Lateral epicondyle
      (8) Trochlea
      (9) Capitulum
      (10) Supraspinatus fossa
      (11) Infraspinatus fossa
      (12) Spine of the scapula
   b. **Subject**
      (1) Shaft
      (2) Medial epicondyle
      (3) Lateral epicondyle
2. How and where do you palpate the following muscles on a human subject?
   a. Deltoid
   b. Teres major
   c. Infraspinatus
   d. Teres minor
   e. Latissimus dorsi
   f. Pectoralis major (upper and lower fibers)
      NOTE: Using the pectoralis major muscle, indicate how various actions allow muscle palpation.
3. Demonstrate and locate on a human subject the muscles that are primarily used in the following shoulder joint movements:
   a. Abduction
   b. Adduction
   c. Flexion
   d. Extension
   e. Horizontal adduction
   f. Horizontal abduction
   g. External rotation
   h. Internal rotation
4. Why is it essential that both anterior and posterior muscles of the shoulder joint be properly developed? What are some activities or sports that would cause unequal development? Equal development?
5. Analyze movements and muscles in both shoulder girdle and shoulder joints when the following activities are performed:
   a. Chinning (actual pull)
   b. Throwing a baseball (throw only)
   c. Batting a baseball (striking ball)
   d. Push up (actual push)
6. Fill in the movements and muscle actions of the shoulder girdle and shoulder joint on the chart at right. List the muscles primarily responsible for each movement.

Muscle analysis chart • Shoulder girdle and shoulder joint

Shoulder girdle	Shoulder joint
Adduction	Extension
Abduction	Flexion
Elevation	Horizontal adduction
Depression	Horizontal abduction
Upward rotation	Abduction
Downward rotation	Adduction
	Outward rotation
	Inward rotation

References

Daniels L, Worthingham C: Muscle testing: techniques of manual examination, ed 5, Philadelphia, 1986, Saunders.

Garth WP, et al: Occult anterior subluxations of the shoulder in noncontact sports, American Journal of Sports Medicine 15:579, November-December 1987.

Lehmkuhl LD, Smith LK: Brunnstrom's clinical kinesiology, ed 4, 1983, Philadelphia, Davis.

Rasch PJ: Kinesiology and applied anatomy, ed 7, Philadelphia, 1989, Lea & Febiger.

Sieg KW, Adams SP: Illustrated essentials of musculoskeletal anatomy, ed 2, Gainesville, Fl, 1985, Megabooks.

Stacey E: Pitching injuries to the shoulder, Athletic Journal 65:44, January 1984.

The elbow and radioulnar joints

Objectives

• **To identify on a human skeleton the most important bone features of the elbow and radioulnar joints.**

• **To label the important bone features on a skeletal chart.**

• **To draw and label the muscles on a skeletal chart.**

• **To palpate the muscles on a human subject.**

• **To organize and list the muscles that produce the primary movements of the elbow joint and the radioulnar joint.**

Practically any movement of the upper extremity will involve the elbow and radioulnar joints. Quite often, these joints are grouped together because of their close anatomical relationship. For this reason, novice students may confuse motions of the elbow with those of the radioulnar joint. In addition, radioulnar joint motion may be incorrectly attributed to the wrist joint because it appears to occur there. However, with close inspection, the elbow joint and its movements may be clearly distinguished from those of the radioulnar joints, just as the radioulnar movements may be distinguished from those of the wrist.

Bones FIG. 4-1

The scapula and humerus serve as the proximal attachments for the muscles that flex and extend the elbow. The ulna and radius serve as the distal attachments for these same muscles. The scapula, humerus, and ulna serve as proximal attachments for the muscles that pronate and supinate the radioulnar joints. The distal attachments of the radioulnar joint muscles are located on the radius.

Joints FIG. 4-1

The elbow joint is classified as a ginglymus or hinge-type joint that allows only flexion and extension. Elbow motions involve primarily movement between the articular surfaces of the humerus and ulna, specifically the humeral trochlea fitting in to the trochlea notch of the ulna. The head of the radius has a relatively small amount of contact with the capitulum of the humerus. As the elbow reaches full extension, the olecranon process of the ulna is received by the olecranon fossa of the humerus. This arrangement provides increased joint stability when the elbow is in full extension.

As the elbow flexes approximately 20 degrees or more, its bony stability is somewhat unlocked, allowing for more side-to-side laxity. The stability of the elbow in flexion is more dependent on the collateral ligaments such as the lateral or radial collateral ligament and especially the medial or ulnar collateral ligament.

The elbow is capable of moving from 0 degrees of extension to approximately 145 to 150 degrees of flexion.

The radioulnar joint is classified as a trochoid or pivot-type joint. The radial head rotates around in its location at the proximal ulna. This rotary movement is accompanied by the distal radius rotating around the distal ulna. The radial head is maintained in its joint by the annular ligament. The radioulnar joint can supinate approximately 80 to 90 degrees from the neutral position. Pronation varies from 70 to 90 degrees.

FIG. 4-1 • Elbow joint. **A,** Anterior view; **B,** lateral view; **C,** medial view.

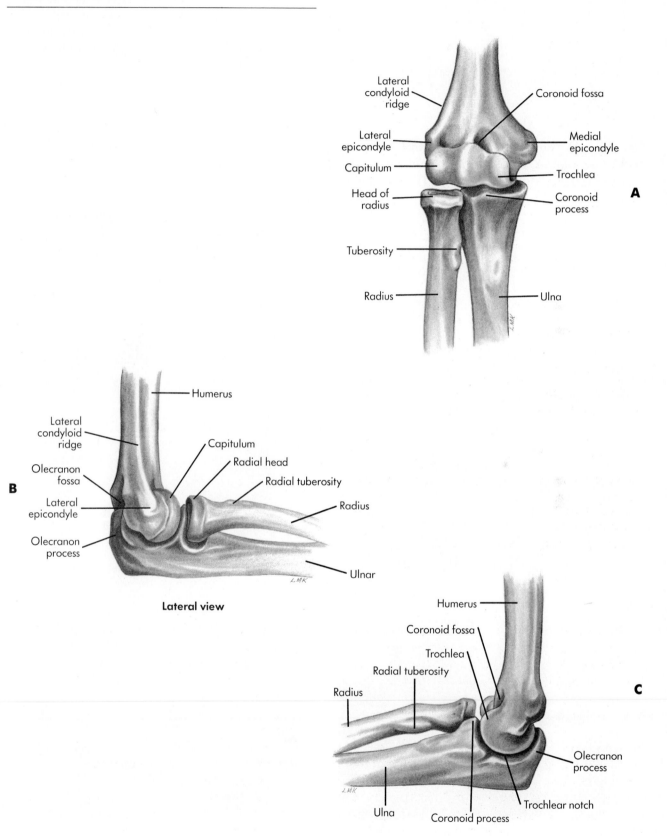

Lateral condyloid ridge

Coronoid fossa

Lateral epicondyle

Medial epicondyle

Capitulum

Trochlea

Head of radius

Coronoid process

Tuberosity

Radius

Ulna

A

Humerus

Lateral condyloid ridge

Capitulum

Radial head

Radial tuberosity

Olecranon fossa

Radius

Lateral epicondyle

Olecranon process

Ulnar

B

Lateral view

Humerus

Coronoid fossa

Trochlea

Radial tuberosity

Radius

C

Olecranon process

Ulna

Coronoid process

Trochlear notch

Flexion: movement of the forearm to the shoulder by bending the elbow to decrease its angle.

Extension: movement of the forearm away from the shoulder by straightening the elbow to increase its angle.

Pronation: internal rotary movement of the radius on the ulna that results in the hand moving from the palm-up to the palm-down position.

Supination: external rotary movement of the radius on the ulna that results in the hand moving from the palm-down to the palm-up position.

FIG. 4-2 • Movements of the elbow and radioulnar joint. **A**, Elbow flexion; **B**, elbow extension; **C**, radioulnar pronation; **D**, radioulnar supination.

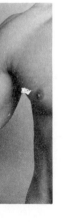

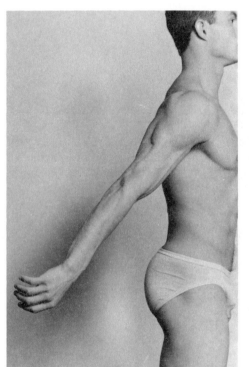

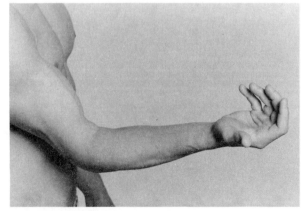

Muscles FIGS. 4-3 and 4-4

The muscles of the elbow and radioulnar joints may be more clearly understood when separated by function. Of the four movements, there are three muscles involved in each, except for extension, in which only two muscles are involved. The elbow flexors are the biceps brachii, the brachialis, and the brachioradialis. The triceps brachii is the primary elbow extensor, with assistance provided by the anconeus. The pronator group consists of the pronator teres, the pronator quadratus, and the brachioradialis. The brachioradialis also assists with supination, which is mainly controlled by the supinator muscle and the biceps brachii.

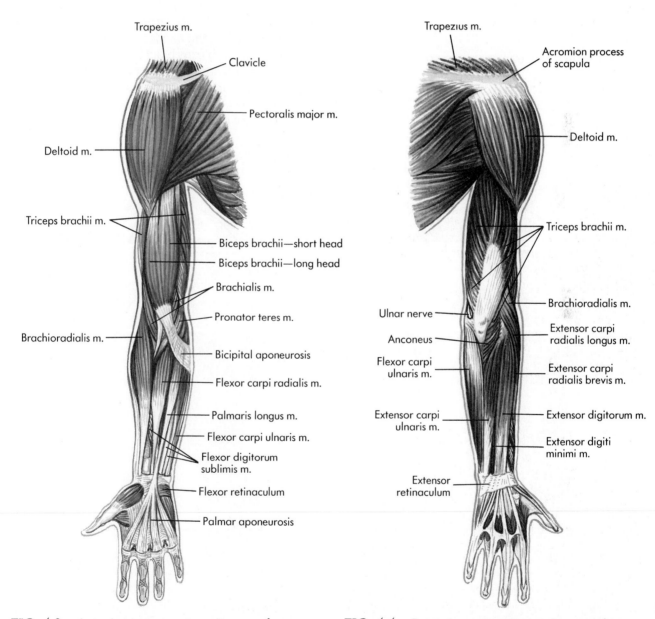

FIG. 4-3 • Anterior upper extremity muscles.

FIG. 4-4 • Posterior upper extremity muscles.

Modified from Thibodeau GA: Anatomy and physiology, St. Louis, 1987, Mosby.

Modified from Thibodeau GA: Anatomy and physiology, St. Louis, 1987, Mosby.

49

Biceps brachii muscle FIG. 4-5

(bi'seps bra'ki-i)

Origin

Two heads

Long head: supraglenoid tubercle above the superior lip of the glenoid fossa.

Short head: coracoid process of the scapula and upper lip of the glenoid fossa.

Insertion

Tuberosity of the radius.

Action

Flexion of the elbow.

Supination of the forearm.

Weak flexion of the shoulder joint.

Palpation

Easily palpated on the anterior aspect of the humerus and elbow.

Innervation

Musculocutaneous nerve (C5,6).

Functional application and strengthening

The biceps is a two-joint (shoulder and elbow) or biarticular muscle. Some authorities consider it to be a three-joint (multiarticular) muscle—shoulder, elbow, and radioulnar. It is weak in actions of the shoulder joint, although it does assist in providing dynamic anterior stability to maintain the humeral head in the glenoid fossa. It is the most powerful flexor of the elbow, especially when the radioulnar joint is supinated. It is a strong supinator, particularly if the elbow is flexed. Palms away from the face (pronation) decrease the effectiveness of the biceps, partly as a result of the disadvantageous pull of the muscle as the radius rotates. The same muscles are used in elbow joint flexion, whether it is pronated or supinated.

Flexion of the forearm, known as "curling," with a barbell in the hands is an excellent exercise to develop the biceps brachii. This movement can be performed one arm at a time with dumbbells or both arms simultaneously with a barbell. Other activities in which there is powerful flexion of the forearm are chinning and rope climbing.

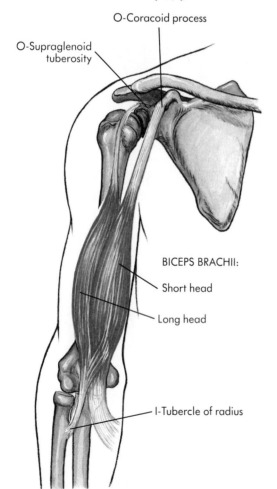
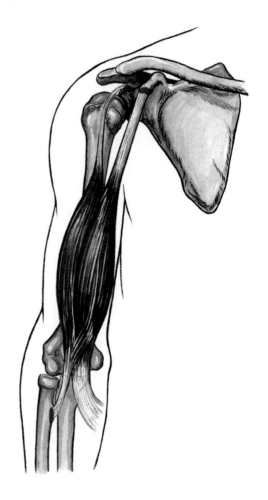

O-Coracoid process

O-Supraglenoid tuberosity

BICEPS BRACHII:

Short head

Long head

I-Tubercle of radius

FIG. 4-5 • Biceps brachii muscle. *O,* Origin; *I,* insertion.

Modified from Thibodeau GA, Patton KT: Anatomy and physiology, ed 2, St. Louis, 1993, Mosby.

Brachialis muscle FIG. 4-6

(bra′ki-a′lis)

Origin

Distal half of the anterior portion of the humerus.

Insertion

Coronoid process and tuberosity of the ulna.

Action

True flexion of the elbow.

Palpation

Lateral side of the upper arm under the biceps brachii muscle.

Innervation

Musculocutaneous nerve and sometimes branches from radial and median nerve (C5,6).

Functional application and strengthening

The brachialis muscle is used along with other flexor muscles, whether in pronation or supination. It pulls on the ulna, which does not rotate, thus making this muscle the only pure flexor of this joint.

The brachialis muscle is called into action whenever the elbow flexes. It is exercised along with elbow curling exercises as described for the biceps brachii, pronator teres, and brachioradialis muscles.

FIG. 4-6 • Brachialis muscle. *O,* Origin; *I,* insertion.

Modified from Anthony CP, Kolthoff NJ: Textbook of anatomy and physiology, ed 9, St. Louis, 1975, Mosby.

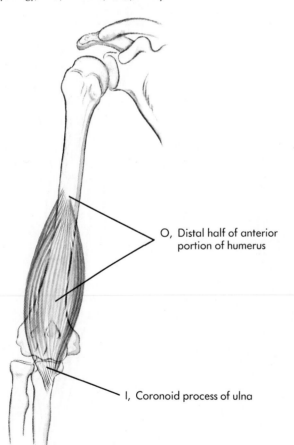

O, Distal half of anterior portion of humerus

I, Coronoid process of ulna

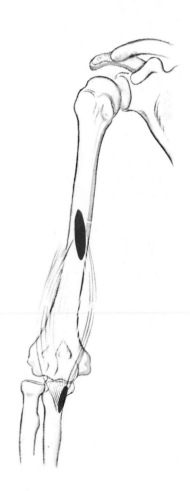

Brachioradialis muscle FIG. 4-7

(bra'ki-o-ra'di-a'lis)

Origin

Distal two thirds of the lateral condyloid (supra-condylar) ridge of the humerus.

Insertion

Lateral surface of the distal end of the radius at the styloid process.

Action

Flexion of the elbow.
Pronation from supinated position to neutral.
Supination from pronated position to neutral.

Palpation

On the lateral anterior side of the forearm.

Innervation

Radial nerve (C5,6).

Functional application and strengthening

The brachioradialis muscle acts as a flexor best in a midposition between pronation and supination. In a supinated position of the forearm, it tends to pronate as it flexes. In a pronated position, it tends to supinate as it flexes. This muscle is favored in its action of flexion when the midposition between pronation and supination is assumed, as previously suggested. Its insertion at the end of the radius makes it a strong elbow flexor. Its ability as a supinator decreases as the radioulnar joint moves toward neutral. Similarly, its ability to pronate decreases as the forearm reaches neutral.

The brachioradialis may be strengthened by performing elbow curls against resistance, particularly with the radioulnar joint in a neutral position. In addition, it may be developed by performing pronation and supination movements through the full range of motion against resistance.

FIG. 4-7 • Brachioradialis muscle. *O,* Origin; *I,* insertion.

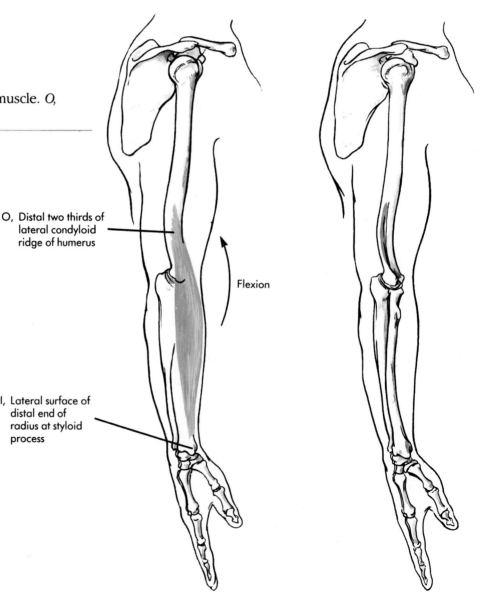

O, Distal two thirds of lateral condyloid ridge of humerus

Flexion

I, Lateral surface of distal end of radius at styloid process

Triceps brachii muscle FIG. 4-8

(tri'seps bra'ki-i)

Origin

Long head: infraglenoid tubercle below inferior lip of glenoid fossa of the scapula.
Lateral head: upper half of the posterior surface of the humerus.
Medial head: distal two thirds of the posterior surface of the humerus.

Insertion

Olecranon process of the ulna.

Action

All heads: extension of the elbow.
Long head: extension of the shoulder joint.

Palpation

Posterior and lateral aspects of the humerus.

Innervation

Radial nerve (C7,8).

Functional application and strengthening

Typical action of the triceps brachii is shown in push-ups when there is powerful extension of the elbow. It is used in hand balancing or in any pushing movement involving the upper extremity. The long head is an important extensor of the shoulder joint.

Two muscles extend the elbow—the triceps brachii and the anconeus. Push-ups demand strenuous contraction of these muscles. Dips on the parallel bars are more difficult to perform. Bench-pressing a barbell or dumbbell upward with weights is an excellent exercise. Overhead presses and french curls or triceps curls emphasize the triceps.

FIG. 4-8 • Triceps brachii muscle. *O,* Origin; *I,* insertion.

Modified from Anthony CP, Kolthoff NJ: Textbook of anatomy and physiology, ed 9, St. Louis, 1975, Mosby.

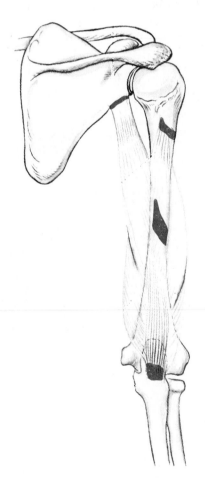

O, Long head—infraglenoid tubercle scapula

O, Lateral head—upper half of posterior surface of humerus

O, Medial head—distal two thirds of posterior surface of humerus

I, Olecranon process of ulna

Anconeus muscle FIG. 4-9

(an-ko'ne-us)

Origin

Posterior surface of the lateral condyle of the humerus.

Insertion

Posterior surface of the olecranon process of the ulna.

Action

Extension of the elbow.

Palpation

Posterior lateral aspect of the olecranon process.

Innervation

Radial nerve (C7,8).

Functional application and strengthening

The chief function of the anconeus muscle is to pull the synovial membrane of the elbow joint out of the way of the advancing olecranon process during extension of the elbow. It contracts along with the triceps brachii. It is strengthened with any elbow extension exercise against resistance.

FIG. 4-9 • Anconeus muscle. *O,* Origin; *I,* insertion.

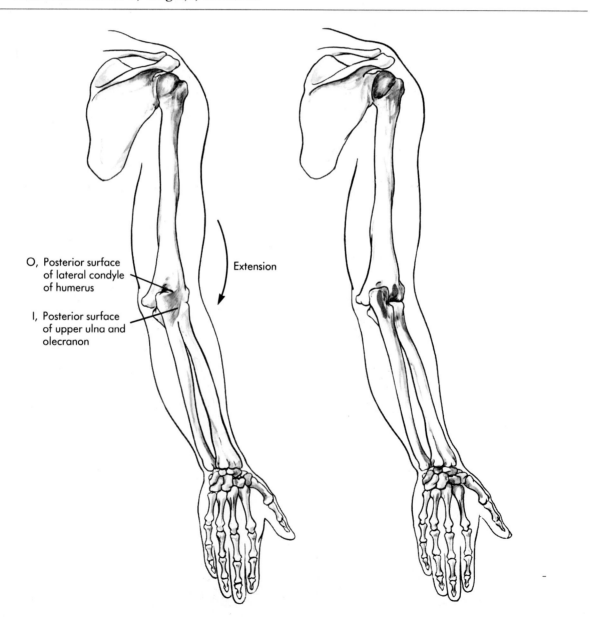

O, Posterior surface of lateral condyle of humerus

I, Posterior surface of upper ulna and olecranon

Extension

Supinator muscle FIG. 4-10

(su′pi-na′tor)

Origin

Lateral condyloid ridge of the humerus and neighboring posterior part of the ulna.

Insertion

Lateral surface of the proximal radius just below the head.

Action

Supination of the elbow.

Palpation

Cannot be palpated.

Innervation

Radial nerve (C6).

Functional application and strengthening

The supinator muscle is called into play when the movements of extension and supination are required, such as turning a screwdriver. The curve in throwing a baseball calls this muscle into play as the elbow is extended just before ball release. Its best development takes place in movements that require supination with elbow extension, because the biceps brachii assist with most supination when the elbow is flexed.

The hands should be grasped, and the forearm extended, in an attempt to supinate the forearms against the grip of the hands. This localizes, to a degree, the action of the supinator.

Strengthening this muscle begins with holding a hammer in the hand with the hammer head suspended from the ulnar side of the hand while the forearm is supported on a desk or table. The hammer should be hanging toward the floor, and the forearm supinated to the palm-up position.

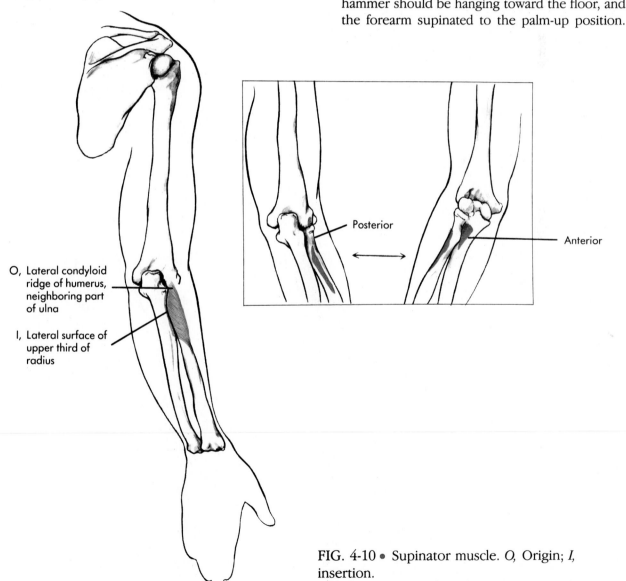

O, Lateral condyloid ridge of humerus, neighboring part of ulna

I, Lateral surface of upper third of radius

Posterior

Anterior

FIG. 4-10 • Supinator muscle. *O,* Origin; *I,* insertion.

Pronator teres muscle FIG. 4-11

(pro-na'tor te'rez)

Origin

Distal part of the medial condyloid ridge of the humerus and medial side of the ulna.

Insertion

Middle third of the lateral surface of the radius.

Action

Pronation of the forearm.
Weak flexion of the elbow.

Palpation

Anteromedial surface of the proximal forearm.

Innervation

Median nerve (C6,7).

Functional application and strengthening

Typical movement of the pronator teres muscle is with the forearm pronating as it flexes. Movement is weaker in flexion with supination. The use of the pronator teres alone in movement tends to bring the back of the hand to the face as it contracts. Pronation of the forearm with a dumbbell in the hand localizes action and develops the pronator teres muscle. The hammer exercise used for the supinator muscle may be modified to develop the pronator teres. In the beginning the forearm is supported, and the hand is free off the table edge. The hammer is again held suspended out of the ulnar side of the hand hanging toward the floor. The forearm is then pronated to the palm-down position to strengthen this muscle.

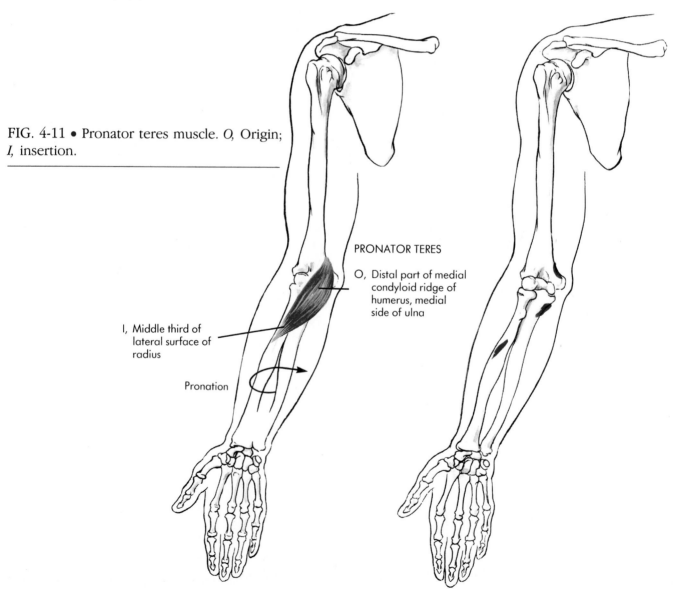

FIG. 4-11 • Pronator teres muscle. *O,* Origin; *I,* insertion.

PRONATOR TERES

O, Distal part of medial condyloid ridge of humerus, medial side of ulna

I, Middle third of lateral surface of radius

Pronation

Pronator quadratus muscle FIG. 4-12
(pro-na'tor kwad-ra'tus)

Origin

Distal fourth of the anterior side of the ulna.

Insertion

Distal fourth of the anterior side of the radius.

Action

Pronation of the forearm.

Palpation

Cannot be palpated.

Innervation

Median nerve (palmar interosseous branch) (C6,7).

Functional application and strengthening

The pronator quadratus muscle works with the triceps brachii muscle in the combined movement of extension and pronation. It is commonly used in turning a screwdriver, when extension and pronation are needed, such as in taking out a screw. It is used also in throwing a screwball, when extension and pronation are needed. It may be developed with similar pronation exercises against resistance as described for the pronator teres.

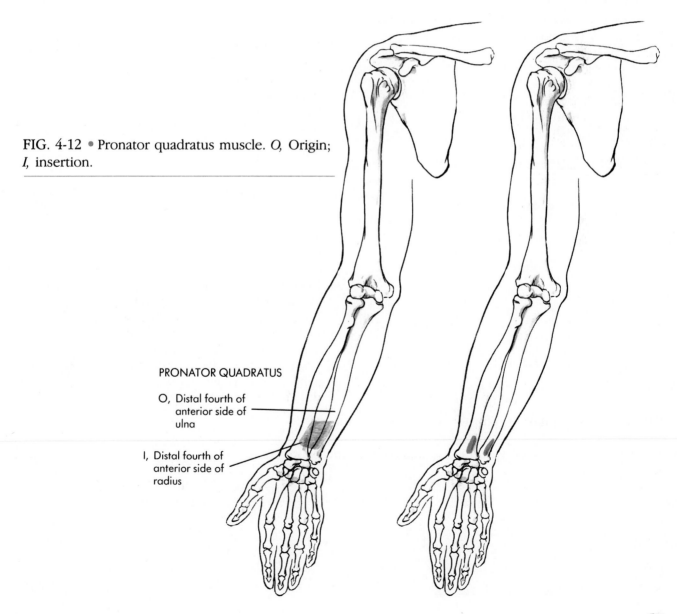

FIG. 4-12 • Pronator quadratus muscle. *O,* Origin; *I,* insertion.

PRONATOR QUADRATUS

O, Distal fourth of anterior side of ulna

I, Distal fourth of anterior side of radius

Worksheet exercises

As an aid to learning, for in-class and out-of-class assignments, or for testing, tearout worksheets are found at the end of the text (p. 219).

Skeletal worksheet (no. 1)

Draw and label on the worksheet the following muscles:
a. Biceps brachii
b. Brachioradialis
c. Brachialis.
d. Pronator teres.
e. Pronator quadratus.
f. Supinator.
g. Triceps brachii.
h. Anconeus

Human figure worksheet (no. 3)

Label and indicate by arrows the following movements of the elbow and radioulnar joints:
1. Elbow joint
   a. Flexion
   b. Extension
2. Radioulnar joint
   a. Pronation
   b. Supination

Laboratory and review exercises

1. Locate the following parts of the humerus, radius, and ulna on a human skeleton and on a subject.
   a. **Skeleton**
      (1) Medial epicondyle
      (2) Lateral epicondyle
      (3) Trochlea
      (4) Capitulum
      (5) Olecranon fossa
      (6) Olecranon process
      (7) Coronoid process
      (8) Coronoid fossa
      (9) Tuberosity of the radius
      (10) Styloid process—radius
      (11) Styloid process—ulna
   b. **Subject**
      (1) Medial epicondyle
      (2) Lateral epicondyle
      (3) Olecranon process
      (4) Olecranon fossa
2. How and where do you palpate the following muscles on a human subject?
   a. Biceps brachii
   b. Brachioradialis
   c. Brachialis
   d. Pronator teres
   e. Supinator
   f. Triceps brachii
   g. Anconeus
3. Palpate and list the muscles primarily responsible for the following movements as you demonstrate each:
   a. Flexion
   b. Extension
   c. Pronation
   d. Supination
4. Discuss the difference in chinning with the palms toward the face and with the palms away from the face. Consider this muscularly and anatomically.
5. How would you ensure proper develoment of the antagonistic muscles at the elbow joint?
6. Fill in the movements and muscle actions of the elbow joint on the following chart. List the muscles primarily responsible for each movement.

Muscle analysis chart • Elbow and radioulnar joints

Elbow and radioulnar joints	
Flexion	Extension
Pronation	Supination

References

Back BR Jr, et al: Triceps rupture: a case report and literature review, American Journal of Sports Medicine 15:285, May-June 1987.

Daniels L, Worthingham C: Muscle testing: techniques of manual examination, ed 5, Philadelphia, 1986, Saunders.

Gabbard CP, et al: Effects of grip and forearm position on flex arm hang performance, Research Quarterly for Exercise and Sport, July 1983.

Herrick RT, Herrick S: Ruptured triceps in powerlifter presenting as cubital tunnel syndrome—a case report, American Journal of Sports Medicine 15:514, September-October 1987.

Lehmkuhl LD, Smith LK: Brunnstrom's clinical kinesiology, ed 4, Philadelphia, 1983, Davis.

Rasch PJ: Kinesiology and applied anatomy, ed 7, Philadelphia, 1989, Lea & Febiger.

Sieg KW, Adams SP: Illustrated essentials of musculoskeletal anatomy, ed 2, Gainesville, Fl, 1985, Megabooks.

Sisto DJ, et al: An electromyographic analysis of the elbow in pitching, American Journal of Sports Medicine 15:260, May-June, 1987.

Springer SI: Racquetball and elbow injuries, National Racquetball 16:7, March 1987.

The wrist and hand joints

Objectives

• To identify on a human skeleton the most important bony features of the wrist, hand, and fingers.

• To label the important bony features on a skeletal chart.

• To draw and label the muscles on a skeletal chart.

• To palpate the muscles on a human subject while demonstrating their actions.

• To organize and list the muscles that produce the primary movements of the wrist, hand, and fingers.

The joints of the wrist, hand, and fingers are often taken for granted. Even though the fine motor skills characteristic of this area are not essential in some sports, many sports with skilled activities require precise functioning of the wrist and hand. Several sports such as archery, bowling, golf, baseball, and tennis require the combined use of all of these joints.

Because of their numerous muscles, bones, and ligaments, combined with their relatively small joint size, the wrist and hand appear to be quite complex. This complexity may be simplified by relating the functional anatomy to the major actions of the joints: flexion, extension, abduction, and adduction of the wrist and hand.

A large number of muscles are used in these movements. Anatomically and structurally, the human wrist and hand have highly developed, complex mechanisms capable of a variety of movements, which is a result of the arrangement of the 29 bones, more than 25 joints, and more than 30 muscles, of which 15 are intrinsic (both origin and insertion found inside the hand) muscles.

For most students who use this text, an extensive knowledge of these intrinsic muscles is not necessary. Athletic trainers, physical therapists, occupational therapists, chiropractors, anatomists, physicians, and nurses require a more extensive knowledge. References at the end of this chapter provide additional sources from which this information can be secured.

Our discussion is limited to a review of the muscles, joints, and movements involved in gross motor activities. The muscles included are those of the forearm and the extrinsic muscles of the wrist, hand, and fingers. The larger, more important extrinsic muscles of each joint are included, providing a limited knowledge of this area. The prescription of exercises for strengthening these muscles will be somewhat redundant, since there are primarily only four movements accomplished by their combined actions. Fingertip push-ups will exercise most of these muscles.

Bones FIG. 5-1

The wrist and hand contain 29 bones, including the radius and ulna. Eight carpal bones in two rows of four bones form the wrist. Five metacarpal bones, numbered one to five from the thumb to the little finger, join the wrist bones. There are 14 phalanges (digits), three for each phalange except the thumb, which has only two. They are indicated as proximal, middle, and distal from the metacarpals.

Joints FIG. 5-1

The wrist joint is classified as a condyloid-type joint, allowing flexion, extension, abduction, and adduction. Wrist motion occurs primarily between the distal radius and the proximal carpal row consisting of the scaphoid, lunate, and triquetrum. The joint allows 70 to 90 degrees of flexion and 65 to 85 degrees of extension. The wrist can abduct 15 to 25 degrees and adduct 25 to 40 degrees.

Each finger has three joints. The metacarpophalangeal joints are classified as condyloid. In these joints, 0 to 40 degrees of extension and 85 to 100 degrees of flexion are possible. The proximal interphalangeal joints, classified as ginglymus, can move from full extension to approximately 90 to 120 degrees of flexion.

The distal interphalangeal joints, also classified as ginglymus, can flex 80 to 90 degrees from full extension.

The thumb has only two joints, both of which are classified as ginglymus. The metacarpophalangeal joint moves from full extension into 40 to 90 degrees of flexion. The interphalangeal joint can flex 80 to 90 degrees. The carpometacarpal joint of the thumb is a unique saddle-type joint having 50 to 70 degrees of abduction. It can flex approximately 15 to 45 degrees and extends 0 to 20 degrees.

Ligaments, too numerous to mention in this discussion, support and provide static stability to the many joints of the wrist and hand.

FIG. 5-1 • Right wrist and hand, palmar surface.

From Anthony CP, Kolthoff NJ: Textbook of anatomy and physiology, ed 9, St. Louis, 1975, Mosby.

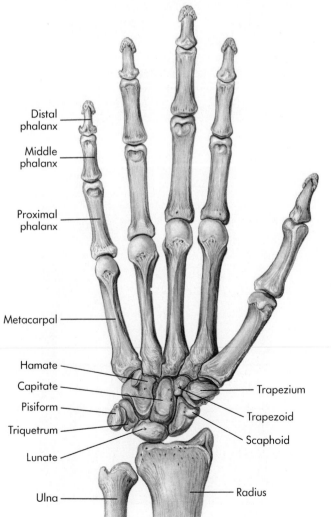

Distal phalanx
Middle phalanx
Proximal phalanx
Metacarpal
Hamate
Capitate
Pisiform
Triquetrum
Lunate
Ulna
Trapezium
Trapezoid
Scaphoid
Radius

Movements FIG. 5-2

The common actions of the wrist are flexion, extension, abduction, and adduction. The fingers can only flex and extend, except at the metacarpophalangeal joints, where abduction and adduction are controlled by the intrinsic hand muscles. These movements, together with pronation and supination of the forearm, make possible the many fine coordinated movements of the forearm, wrist, and hand.

Flexion: moving the palm of the hand and/or phalanges toward the anterior or volar aspect of the forearm.

Extension: moving the back of the hand and/or phalanges toward the posterior or dorsal aspect of the forearm.

Abduction: (radial flexion) movement of the thumb side of the hand toward the lateral aspect or radial side of the forearm.

Adduction: (ulnar flexion) movement of the little finger side of the hand toward the medial aspect or ulnar side of the forearm.

Opposition: movement of the thumb across the palmar aspect to oppose any or all of the phalanges.

FIG. 5-2 • Wrist and hand movements. **A,** Wrist flexion; **B,** wrist extension; **C,** wrist abduction; **D,** wrist adduction.

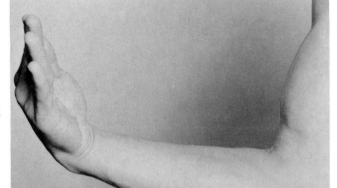

A

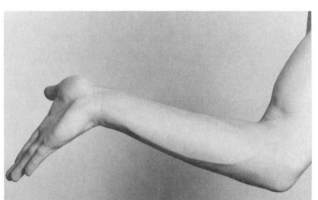

B

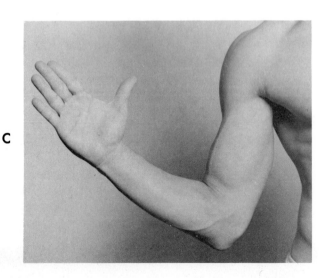

C

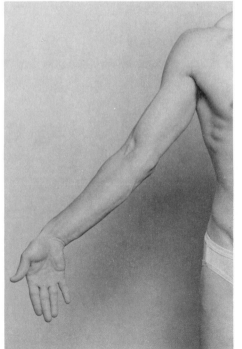

D

Muscles

The extrinsic muscles of the wrist and hand may be grouped according to function and location. There are six muscles that move the wrist but do not cross the hand to move the fingers and thumb. The three wrist flexors in this group include the flexor carpi radialis, flexor carpi ulnaris, and palmaris longus. The extensor carpi radialis longus, extensor carpi radialis brevis, and extensor carpi ulnaris are the wrist extensors in this group.

There are another nine muscles that function primarily to move the phalanges but are also involved in wrist joint actions because they originate on the forearm and cross the wrist. These muscles generally are weaker in their actions on the wrist. The flexor digitorum superficialis and the flexor digitorum profundus are finger flexors; but they also assist in wrist flexion along with the flexor pollicis longus, which is a thumb flexor. The extensor digitorum, the extensor indicis, and the extensor digiti minimi are finger extensors but also assist in wrist extension, along with the extensor pollicis longus and the extensor pollicis brevis,

which extend the thumb. The abductor pollicis longus abducts the thumb and assists in wrist abduction.

All of the wrist flexors generally have their origins on the anteromedial aspect of the proximal forearm and medial epicondyle of the humerus, whereas their insertions are on the anterior aspect of the wrist and hand. The wrist extensors generally have their origins on the posterolateral aspect of the proximal forearm and lateral humeral epicondyle, whereas their insertions are located on the posterior aspect of the wrist and hand. The wrist abductors include the flexor carpi radialis, the extensor carpi radialis longus, the extensor carpi radialis brevis, the abductor pollicis longus, the extensor pollicis longus, and the extensor pollicis brevis. These muscles generally cross the wrist joint anterolaterally and posterolaterally to insert on the radial side of the hand. The flexor carpi ulnaris and extensor carpi ulnaris adduct the wrist and cross the wrist joint anteromedially and posteromedially to insert on the ulnar side of the hand.

FIG. 5-2, cont'd • Wrist and hand movements. **E**, flexion of the fingers and thumb; **F**, extension of the fingers and thumb.

E 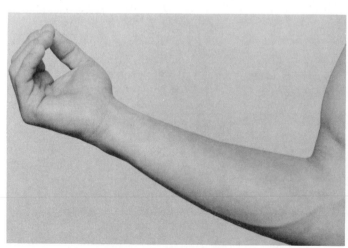 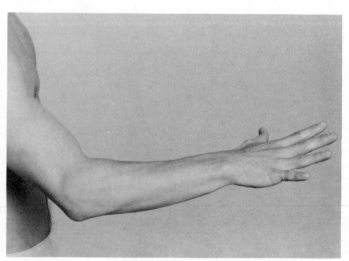 F

Flexor carpi radialis muscle FIG. 5-3

(fleks'or kar'pi ra'di-a'lis)

Origin

Medial epicondyle of the humerus.

Insertion

Base of the second and third metacarpals, anterior (palmar surface).

Action

Flexion of the wrist.
Abduction of wrist
Weak flexion of the elbow.

Palpation

Anterior surface of the wrist, slightly lateral, in line with the second and third metacarpals.

Innervation

Median nerve (C6,7).

Functional application and strengthening

The flexor carpi radialis, along with the flexor carpi ulnaris and the palmaris longus, are the most powerful of the wrist flexors. They are brought into play during any activity that requires wrist curling or stabilization of the wrist against resistance, particularly if the forearm is supinated.

It may be developed by performing wrist curls against a hand-held resistance. This may be accomplished when the supinated forearm is being supported by a table with the hand and wrist hanging over the edge to allow full range of motion. The extended wrist is then flexed or curled up to strengthen this muscle.

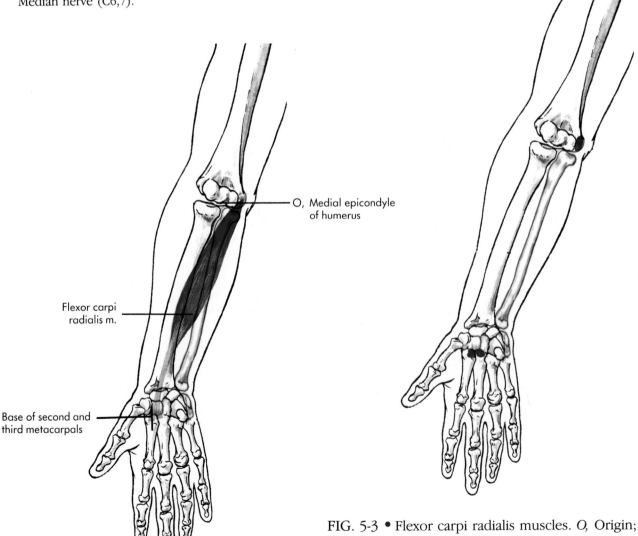

O, Medial epicondyle of humerus

Flexor carpi radialis m.

Base of second and third metacarpals

FIG. 5-3 • Flexor carpi radialis muscles. *O*, Origin; *I*, insertion.

Palmaris longus muscle FIG. 5-4

(pal-ma'ris long'gus)

Origin

Medial epicondyle of the humerus.

Insertion

Palmar aponeurosis of the second, third, fourth, and fifth metacarpals.

Action

Flexion of the wrist.

Palpation

Anterior medial aspect of forearm and anterior centrally just proximal to the wrist.

Innervation

Median nerve (C6,7).

Functional application and strengthening

Unlike the flexor carpi radialis and flexor carpi ulnaris, which are not only wrist flexors, but also abductors and adductors, respectively, the palmaris longus is involved only in wrist flexion because of its central location on the anterior forearm and wrist. It may also be strengthened with any type of wrist-curling activity such as the ones described for the flexor carpi radialis muscle.

FIG. 5-4 • Palmaris longus muscle. *O,* Origin; *I,* insertion.

Modified from Thibodeau GA, Patton KT: Anatomy and physiology, St. Louis, 1993, Mosby.

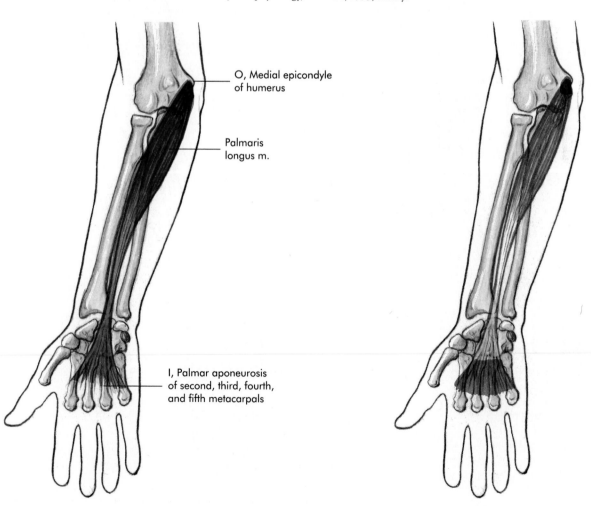

O, Medial epicondyle of humerus

Palmaris longus m.

I, Palmar aponeurosis of second, third, fourth, and fifth metacarpals

Flexor carpi ulnaris muscle FIG. 5-5

(fleks'or kar'pi ul-na'ris)

Origin

Medial epicondyle of the humerus.
Posterior aspect of the proximal ulna.

Insertion

Base of the fifth metacarpal, pisiform, and hamate.

Action

Flexion of the wrist.
Adduction of the wrist, together with the extensor carpi ulnaris muscle.
Weak flexion of the elbow.

Palpation

Anteromedial surface of the forearm, a few inches below the medial epicondyle of the humerus to just proximal to the wrist.

Innervation

Ulnar nerve (C8, T1).

Functional application and strengthening

The flexor carpi ulnaris is very important in wrist flexion or curling activities. In addition, it is one of only two muscles involved in wrist adduction or ulnar flexion. It may be strengthened with any type of wrist curling activity against resistance similar to those described for the flexor carpi radialis muscle.

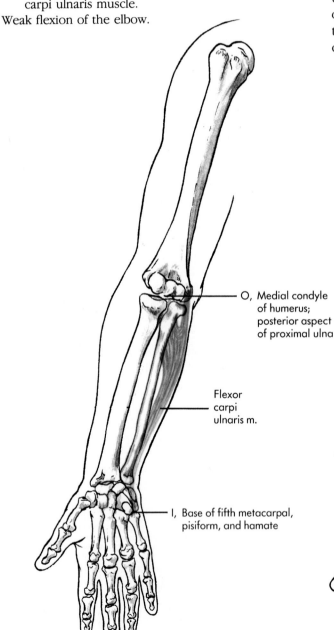

O, Medial condyle of humerus; posterior aspect of proximal ulna

Flexor carpi ulnaris m.

I, Base of fifth metacarpal, pisiform, and hamate

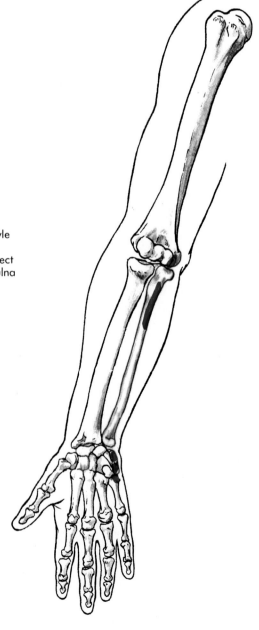

FIG. 5-5 • Flexor carpi ulnaris muscle. *O*, Origin; *I*, insertion.

Extensor carpi ulnaris muscle FIG. 5-6

(eks-ten′sor kar′pi ul-na′ris)

Origin

Lateral epicondyle of the humerus.

Insertion

Base of the fifth metacarpal (dorsal surface).

Action

Extension of the wrist.
Adduction of the wrist together with the flexor carpi
ulnaris muscle.
Weak extension of the forearm.

Palpation

Anterior ulnar side of the forearm near the fifth
metacarpal.

Innervation

Radial nerve (C6,7,8).

Functional application and strengthening

Besides being a powerful wrist extensor, the
extensor carpi ulnaris muscle is the only muscle
other than the flexor carpi ulnaris involved in wrist
adduction or ulnar flexion. Wrist extension exercises such as those described for the extensor
carpi radialis longus are appropriate for development of the muscle.

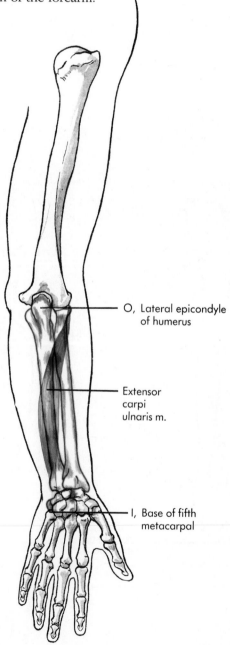

O, Lateral epicondyle
of humerus

Extensor
carpi
ulnaris m.

I, Base of fifth
metacarpal

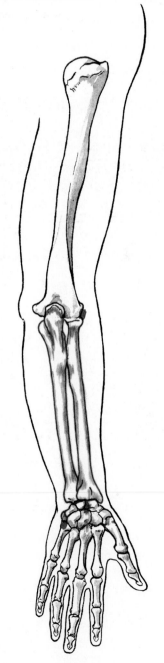

FIG. 5-6 • Extensor carpi ulnaris muscle. *O*,
Origin; *I*, insertion.

Extensor carpi radialis brevis muscle

FIG. 5-7

(eks-ten′sor kar′pi ra′di-a′lis bre′vis)

Origin

Lateral epicondyle of the humerus.

Insertion

Base of the third metacarpal (dorsal surface).

Action

Extension of the wrist.
Abduction of the wrist.
Weak extension of the elbow.

Palpation

Dorsal side of the forearm, which is difficult to palpate.

FIG. 5-7 • Extensor carpi radialis brevis muscle.
O, Origin; I, insertion.

Innervation

Radial nerve (C6,7).

Functional application and strengthening

The extensor carpi radialis brevis, like the extensor carpi radialis longus, is important in any sports activity that requires powerful wrist extension. In addition, both of these muscles are involved in abduction of the wrist. The extensor carpi radialis brevis may be developed with the same wrist extension exercises as described for the extensor carpi radialis longus muscle.

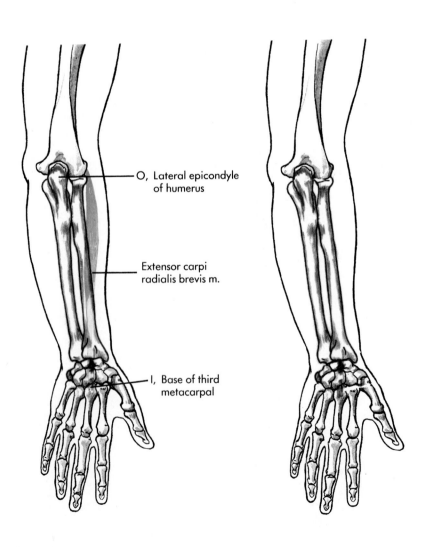

O, Lateral epicondyle of humerus

Extensor carpi radialis brevis m.

I, Base of third metacarpal

Extensor carpi radialis longus muscle FIG. 5-8

(eks-ten′sor kar′pi ra′di-a′lis long′gus)

Origin

Lateral epicondyle of the humerus.

Insertion

Base of the second metacarpal (dorsal surface).

Action

Extension of the wrist.
Abduction of the wrist.
Weak extension of the elbow.

Palpation

Posterior aspect of proximal forearm and anterolateral surface just proximal to the wrist, in line with the second metacarpal.

Innervation

Radial nerve (C6,7).

Functional application and strengthening

The extensor carpi radialis longus, the extensor carpi radialis brevis, and the extensor carpi ulnaris are the most powerful of the wrist extensors. Any activity requiring wrist extension or stabilization of the wrist against resistance, particularly if the forearm is pronated, depends greatly on the strength of these muscles. They are often brought into play with the backhand in racket sports.

The extensor carpi radialis longus may be developed by performing wrist extension against a hand-held resistance. This may be accomplished with the pronated forearm being supported by a table with the hand hanging over the edge to allow full range of motion. The wrist is then moved from the fully flexed position to the fully extended position against the resistance.

FIG. 5-8 • Extensor carpi radialis longus muscle.
O, Origin; *I,* insertion.

Modified from Booher JA, Thibodeau GA: Athletic injury assessment, ed 2, St. Louis, 1989, Mosby.

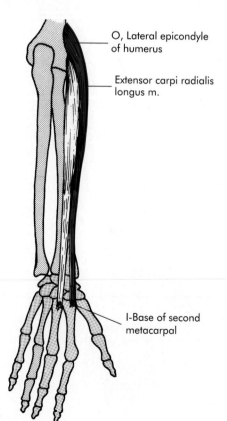

O, Lateral epicondyle of humerus

Extensor carpi radialis longus m.

I-Base of second metacarpal

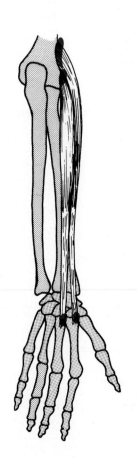

Flexor digitorum superficialis muscle FIG. 5-9

(fleks′or dij-i-to′rum su′per-fish-e-al′is)

Origin

Medial epicondyle of the humerus.
Ulnar head: medial coronoid process.
Radial head: radial tuberosity area and just distally on the anterior radius.

Insertion

Each tendon splits and attaches to the sides of the middle phalanx of four fingers (palmar surface).

Action

Flexion of the fingers.
Flexion of the wrist.
Weak flexion of the elbow.

Palpation

Anterior wrist surface on the ulnar side next to the flexor carpi ulnaris muscle.

Innervation

Median nerve (C7,8 T1).

Functional application and strengthening

The flexor digitorum superficialis muscle, also known as the flexor digitorum sublimis, divides into four tendons on the palmar aspect of the wrist and hand to insert on each of the four fingers. The flexor digitorum superficialis and the flexor digitorum profundus are the only muscles involved in flexion of all four fingers. Both of these muscles are vital in any type of gripping activities.

Squeezing a sponge rubber ball in the palm of the hand, along with other gripping and squeezing activites, can be used to develop these muscles.

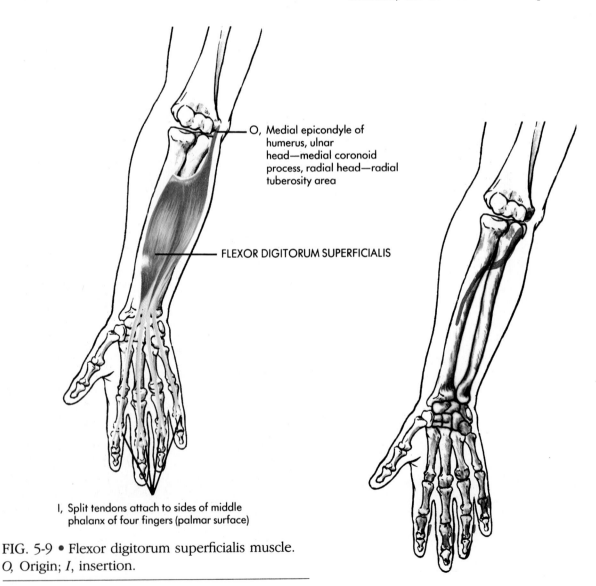

O, Medial epicondyle of humerus, ulnar head—medial coronoid process, radial head—radial tuberosity area

FLEXOR DIGITORUM SUPERFICIALIS

I, Split tendons attach to sides of middle phalanx of four fingers (palmar surface)

FIG. 5-9 • Flexor digitorum superficialis muscle. O, Origin; I, insertion.

Flexor digitorum profundus muscle

FIG. 5-10

(fleks'or dij-i-to'rum pro-fun'dus)

Origin

Proximal three fourths of the anterior and medial ulna.

Insertion

Base of the distal phalanges of the four fingers.

Action

Flexion of the four fingers at the distal interphalangeal joint.
Flexion of the wrist.

Palpation

Anterior surface of middle phalanges of the four fingers.

Innervation

Median nerve (C8, T1) to second and third fingers. Ulnar nerve (C8, T1) to the fourth and fifth fingers.

Functional application and strengthening

Both the flexor digitorum profundus muscle and the flexor digitorum superficialis muscle assist in wrist flexion because of their palmar relationship to the wrist. The flexor digitorum profundus is used in any type of gripping, squeezing, or hand-clenching activity such as gripping a racket or climbing a rope.

The flexor digitorum profundus muscle may be developed through these activities in addition to the strengthening exercises described for the flexor digitorum superficialis muscle.

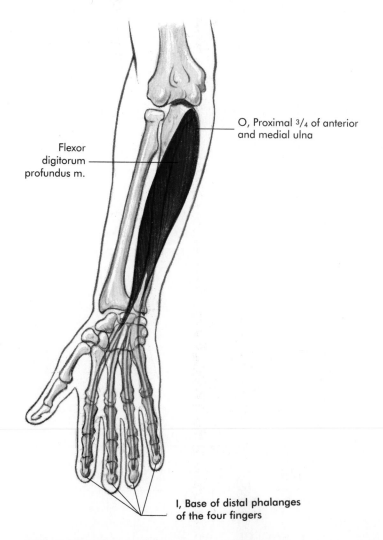
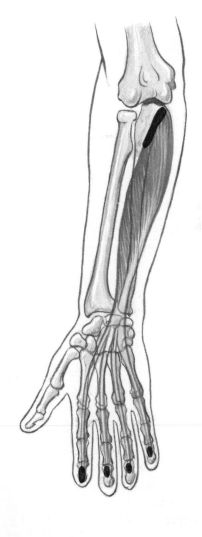

Flexor digitorum profundus m.

O, Proximal 3/4 of anterior and medial ulna

I, Base of distal phalanges of the four fingers

FIG. 5-10 • Flexor digitorum profundus muscle. *O,* Origin; *I,* insertion.

Modified from Thibodeau GA, Patton KT: Anatomy and physiology, ed 2, St. Louis, 1993, Mosby.

Flexor pollicis longus muscle FIG. 5-11

(fleks'or pol'i-sis long'gus)

Origin

Middle anterior surface of the radius.

Insertion

Base of the distal phalanx of the thumb (palmar surface).

Action

Flexion of the thumb.
Flexion of the wrist.

Palpation

Anterior surface of the thumb.

Innervation

Median nerve, palmar interosseous branch (C8,T1).

Functional application and strengthening

The primary function of the flexor pollicis longus muscle is flexion of the thumb, which is vital in gripping and grasping activities of the hand. Because of its palmar relationship to the wrist, it provides some assistance in wrist flexion.

It may be strengthened by squeezing a sponge rubber ball into the hand with the thumb and many other gripping or squeezing activites.

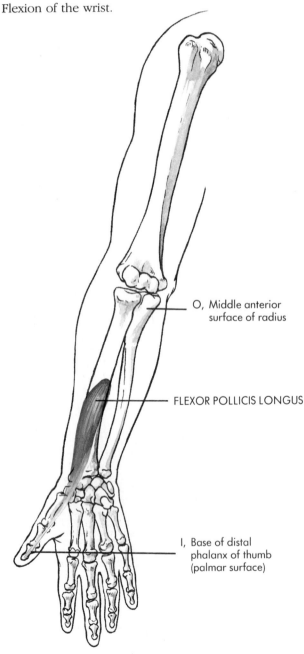

O, Middle anterior surface of radius

FLEXOR POLLICIS LONGUS

I, Base of distal phalanx of thumb (palmar surface)

FIG. 5-11 • Flexor pollicis longus muscle. *O*, Origin; *I*, insertion.

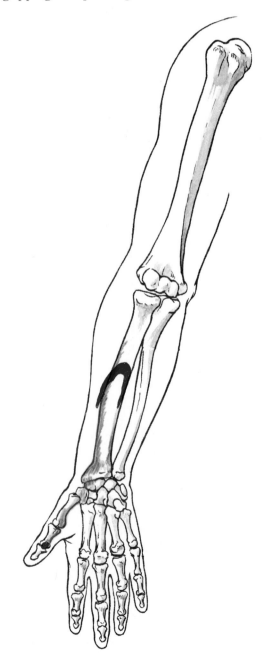

Extensor digitorum muscle FIG. 5-12

(eks-ten'sor dij-i-to'rum)

Origin

Lateral epicondyle of humerus.

Insertion

Four tendons to bases of second and third phalanges of four fingers (dorsal surface).

Action

Extension of the second, third, fourth, and fifth phalanges at the metacarpophalangeal joints. Extension of the wrist. Weak extension of the elbow.

Palpation

Middorsal surface of the forearm and dorsal aspect of the hand.

Innervation

Radial nerve (C6,7,8).

Functional application and strengthening

The extensor digitorum, also know as the extensor digitorum communis, is the only muscle involved in extension of all four fingers. This muscle divides into four tendons on the dorsum of the wrist to insert on each of the fingers. It also assists with wrist extension movements. It may be developed by applying manual resistance to the dorsal aspect of the flexed fingers and then extending the fingers fully. When performed with the wrist in flexion, this exercise increases the workload on the extensor digitorum.

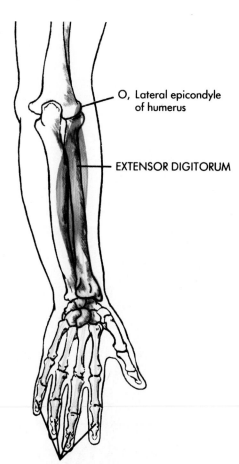

O, Lateral epicondyle of humerus

EXTENSOR DIGITORUM

I, Four tendons to bases of second and third phalanges of four fingers (dorsal surface)

FIG. 5-12 • Extensor digitorum muscle. *O*, Origin; *I*, insertion.

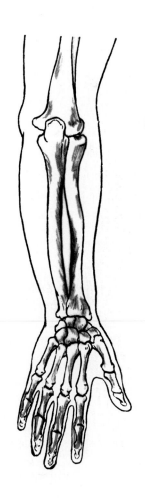

Extensor indicis muscle FIG. 5-13

(eks-ten′sor in′di-sis)

Origin

Middle to distal one third of posterior ulna.

Insertion

Proximal phalanx and extensor expansion of the index finger (dorsal surface).

Action

Extension of the index finger at the metacarpophalangeal joint.

Weak wrist extension.

Palpation

Posterior aspect of the distal forearm and dorsal surface of the hand just medial to the extensor digitorum tendon of the index finger.

Innervation

Radial nerve (C6,7,8).

Functional application and strengthening

The extensor indicis muscle is the pointing muscle. That is, it is responsible for extending the index finger, particularly when the other fingers are flexed. It also provides weak assistance to wrist extension and may be developed through exercises much as those described for the extensor digitorum.

FIG. 5-13 • Extensor indicis muscle. *O,* Origin; *I,* insertion.

Modified from Booher JA, Thibodeau GA: Athletic injury assessment, ed 2, St. Louis, 1989, Mosby.

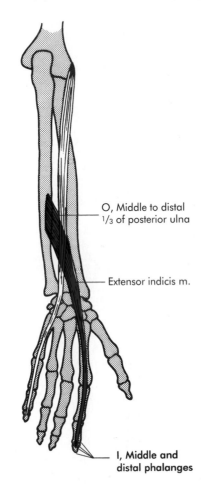

O, Middle to distal
1/3 of posterior ulna

Extensor indicis m.

I, Middle and
distal phalanges

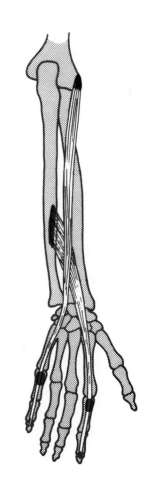

Extensor digiti minimi muscle FIG. 5-14

(eks-ten'sor dij'i-ti min'im-i)

Origin

Lateral epicondyle of humerus.

Insertion

Proximal phalanx of the fifth phalange (dorsal surface).

Action

Extension of the little finger at the metacarpophalangeal joint.

Weak wrist extension.

Palpation

Cannot palpate.

Innervation

Radial nerve (C6,7,8).

Functional application and strengthening

The primary function of the extensor digiti minimi muscle is to assist the extensor digitorum in extending the little finger. Because of its dorsal relationship to the wrist, it also provides weak assistance in wrist extension. It is strengthened with the same exercises as described for the extensor digitorum.

FIG. 5-14 • Extensor digiti minimi muscle. *O,* Origin; *I,* insertion.

Modified from Booher JA, Thibodeau GA: Athletic injury assessment, ed 2, St. Louis, 1989, Mosby.

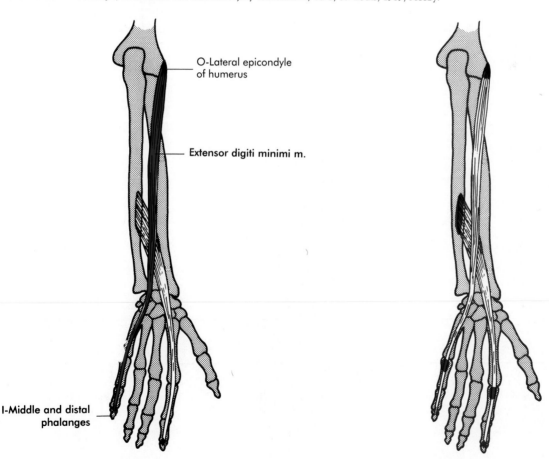

O-Lateral epicondyle of humerus

Extensor digiti minimi m.

I-Middle and distal phalanges

Extensor pollicis longus muscle

FIG. 5-15

(eks-ten′sor pol′i-sis long′gus)

Origin

Upper posterior lateral surface of the ulna.

Insertion

Base of the distal phalanx of the thumb (dorsal surface.)

Action

Extension of the wrist.
Extension of the thumb.

FIG. 5-15 • Extensor pollicis longus muscle. *O*, Origin; *I*, insertion.

Palpation

Most prominent on the dorsal side of the hand.

Innervation

Radial nerve (C6,7,8).

Functional application and strengthening

The primary function of the extensor pollicis longus muscle is extension of the thumb, although it does provide weak assistance in wrist extension.

It may be strengthened by extending the flexed thumb against manual resistance.

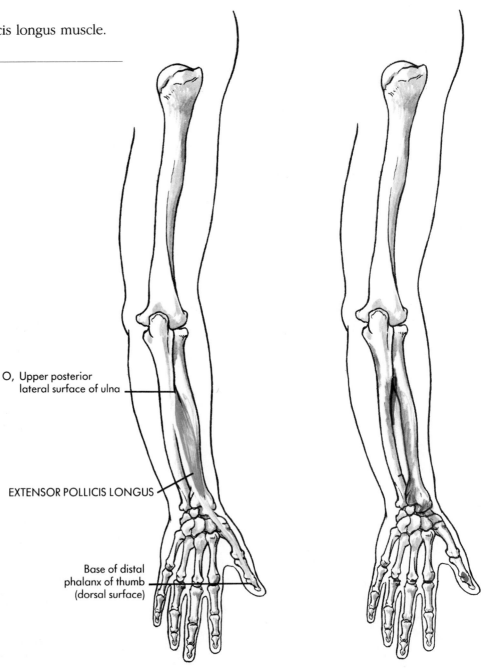

O, Upper posterior lateral surface of ulna

EXTENSOR POLLICIS LONGUS

Base of distal phalanx of thumb (dorsal surface)

Extensor pollicis brevis muscle

FIG. 5-16

(eks-ten'sor pol'i-sis bre'vis)

Origin

Posterior surface of lower middle radius.

Insertion

Base of proximal phalanx of the thumb (dorsal surface).

Action

Extension of the thumb at the metacarpophalangeal joint.

Weak wrist extension.

Palpation

Most prominent on dorsal side of the hand and wrist.

Innervation

Radial nerve (C6,7).

Functional application and strengthening

The extensor pollicis brevis serves to assist the extensor pollicis longus in extending the thumb. Because of its dorsal relationship to the wrist, it too provides weak assistance in wrist extension.

It may be strengthened through the same exercises as described for the extensor pollicis longus muscle.

FIG. 5-16 • Extensor pollicis brevis muscle. *O,* Origin; *I,* insertion.

Modified from Booher JA, Thibodeau GA: Athletic injury assessment, ed 2, St. Louis, 1989, Mosby.

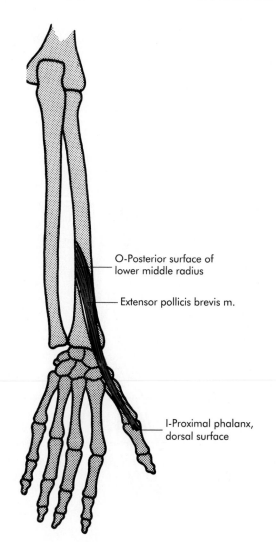

O-Posterior surface of lower middle radius

Extensor pollicis brevis m.

I-Proximal phalanx, dorsal surface

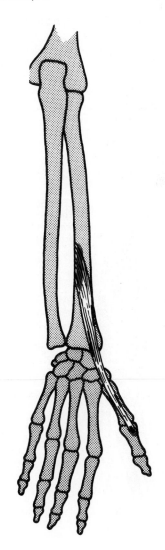

Abductor pollicis longus muscle

FIG. 5-17

(ab-duk'tor pol'i-sis lon'gus)

Origin

Posterior aspect of the radius and midshaft of ulna.

Insertion

Base of the first metacarpal (dorsal surface).

Action

Abduction of the thumb at the carpometacarpal joint. Abduction of the wrist.

Palpation

Lateral aspect of the wrist joint just proximal to the first metacarpal.

Innervation

Radial nerve (C6,7).

Functional application and strengthening

The primary function of the abductor pollicis longus muscle is abduction of the thumb, although it does provide some assistance in abduction of the wrist. It may be developed by abducting the thumb from the adducted position against a manually applied resistance. The abductor pollicis brevis, along with the tendons of the extensor pollicis longus and brevis, forms the anatomical snuffbox.

FIG. 5-17 • Abductor pollicis longus muscle. *O,* Origin; *I,* insertion.

Modified from Booher JA, Thibodeau GA: Athletic injury assessment, ed 2, St. Louis, 1989, Mosby.

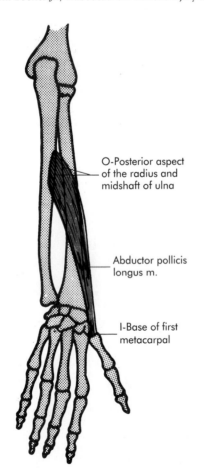

O-Posterior aspect of the radius and midshaft of ulna

Abductor pollicis longus m.

I-Base of first metacarpal

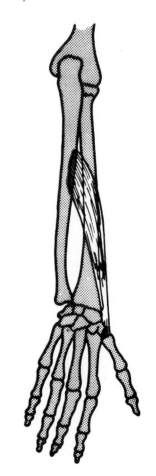

Worksheet exercises

As an aid to learning, for in-class and out-of-class assignments, or for testing, tearout worksheets are found at the end of the text (pp. 220 and 221).

Skeletal worksheet (no.1)

Draw and label on the worksheet the following muscles.
a. Flexor pollicis longus
b. b.Flexor carpi radialis
c. Flexor carpi ulnaris
d. Extensor digitorum
e. Extensor pollicis longus
f. Extensor carpi ulnaris

Human figure worksheet (no. 2)

Label and indicate by arrows the following movements of the wrist and hands:
a. Flexion
b. Extension
c. Abduction (ulnar flexion)
d. Adduction (radial flexion)

Laboratory and review exercises

1. Locate the following parts of the humerus, radius, and ulna on a human skeleton and on a subject:
   a. **Skeleton**
      (1) Medial epicondyle
      (2) Lateral epicondyle
      (3) Trochlea
      (4) Capitulum
      (5) Coronoid process
      (6) Tuberosity of the radius
      (7) Styloid process—radius
      (8) Styloid process—ulna
      (9) First and third metacarpals
      (10) Wrist bones
      (11) First phalanx of third metacarpal
   b. **Subject**
      (1) Medial epicondyle
      (2) Lateral epicondyle
      (3) Pisiform
      (4) Scaphoid (navicular)
2. How and where do you palpate the following muscles on a human subject?
   a. Flexor pollicis longus
   b. Flexor carpi radialis
   c. Flexor carpi ulnaris
   d. Extensor digitorum communis
   e. Extensor pollicis longus
   f. Extensor carpi ulnaris
3. Demonstrate the action and list the muscles primarily responsible for these movements at the wrist joint:
   a. Flexion
   b. Extension
   c. Abduction
   d. Adduction
4. Discuss why the thumb is the most important part of the hand.
5. How should boys and girls be taught to do push-ups? Justify your answer.
   a. Hands flat on floor
   b. Fingertips
6. Fill in the movements and muscle actions of the wrist and hand on the following chart. List the muscles primarily responsible for each movement.

Muscle analysis chart • Wrist, hand, and fingers

Wrist and hand	
Flexion	Extension
Adduction	Abduction
Fingers and thumb	
Flexion	Extension

References

Daniels L, Worthingham C: Muscle testing techniques of manual examination, ed 5, 1989, Philadelphia, Saunders.

Gabbard CP, et al: Effects of grip and forearm position on flex arm hang performance, Res Q Exercise Sport, July 1983.

Herrick RT, Herrick S: Ruptured triceps in powerlifter presenting as cubital tunnel syndrome—a case report, American Journal of Sports Medicine 15:514, September-October 1987.

Lehmkuhl LD, Smith LK: Brunnstrom's clinical kinesiology, ed 4, Philadelphia, 1983, Davis.

Norkin CC, Levangie PK: Joint structure and function—a comprehensive analysis, Philadelphia, 1983, Davis.

Norkin CC, White DJ: Measurement of joint motion: a guide to goniometry, Philadelphia, 1985, Davis.

Sieg KW, Adams SP: Illustrated essentials of musculoskeletal anatomy, ed 2, Gainesville, Fl, 1985, Megabooks.

Sisto DJ, et al: An electromyographic analysis of the elbow in pitching, American Journal of Sports Medicine 15:260, May-June 1987.

Springer SI: Racquetball and elbow injuries, National Racquetball 16:7, March 1987.

Muscular analysis of upper extremities

6

Objectives

- To know and understand the different types of muscle contractions.

- To learn to group individual muscles into units that produce certain joint movements.

- To begin to think of exercises that increase the strength and endurance of individual muscle groups.

- To analyze simple exercises in terms of the joint movements and muscles exercised.

The shoulder areas are the body's weakest area. American boys and girls are extremely weak in the upper shoulder area. A majority are unable to do one chin-up. The traditional chin-up (pull-up) has the subject grasping a horizontal bar with the feet off the floor. The body is then pulled up until the chin is over the bar. The modified chin-up (pull-up) has the feet on the floor; the subject grasps the horizontal bar and pulls the upper body up to touching the bar. The traditional chin up (pull up) had to be modified to secure more meaningful results.*

Strength and endurance in this part of the human body are essential for improved appear-

*Pate R, et al: The national children and youth fitness study. II. The modified pull-up test, Journal of Physical Education, Recreation, and Dance 58:71, 1987.

ance and posture, as well for as more efficient skill performance. Specific exercises and activities to enhance this area should be intelligently selected by becoming thoroughly familiar with the muscles involved.

At this stage, simple exercises are used to begin teaching individuals how to group muscles together to produce joint movement. Some of these simple introductory exercises are included in this chapter.

The early analysis of exercise makes the study of structural kinesiology more meaningful as students come to better understand the importance of individual muscles and groups of muscles in bringing about joint movements in various exercises. Chapter 10 contains a more comprehensive analysis of exercises for all the muscle groups of the entire body. Contrary to what most beginning students in structural kinesiology believe, muscular analysis of activities is not difficult, once the basic concepts are understood.

Concepts for analysis

In analyzing activities, it is important to understand how muscles work together in groups and in paired opposition to perform various joint movements. Students should be able to view an activity and to not only determine which muscles are performing the movement, but also to know the type of contraction that is occurring and what kind of exercises are appropriate for developing the muscles.

Types of muscle contraction

Even though the different types of muscle contractions were defined and explained in Chapter 1, a brief review is included here.

Isometric contraction

Occurs when tension is developed within the muscle but no appreciable change occurs in the joint angle or in the length of the muscle; also known as a static contraction.

Isotonic contraction

Occurs when tension is developed in the muscle while it either shortens or lengthens; also known as a dynamic contraction and may be classified as being either concentric or eccentric.

Concentric contraction

Involves the muscle developing tension as it shortens and occurs when the muscle develops enough force to overcome the applied resistance. Concentric contractions may be thought of as causing movement against gravity or resistance and are described as being positive contractions.

Eccentric contraction

Involves the muscle lengthening under tension and occurs when the muscle gradually lessens in tension to control the descent of the resistance. Eccentric contractions may be thought of as controlling movement with gravity or resistance and are described as negative contractions.

Various exercises may use any one or all of these contraction types for muscle development. Recent development of exercise machines has resulted in another type of muscle exercise known as *isokinetics*. Isokinetics is not another type of contraction, as some authorities have described; rather, it is a specific technique that may use any or all of the different types of contractions. Isokinetics is a type of dynamic exercise usually using concentric and/or eccentric muscle contractions in which the speed (or velocity) of movement is constant and muscular contraction (usually maximum contraction) occurs throughout the movement. Biodex, Cybex, KinCom, Lido, and other new types of apparatuses are engineered to allow this type of exercise.

Students well-educated in kinesiology should be qualified to prescribe exercises and activities for the development of large muscles and muscle groups in the human body. They should be able to read the description of an exercise or observe an exercise and immediately know the most important muscles that are being used. Following are some terms used to describe how muscles function in joint movement.

Agonist

Muscles that cause or control joint motion through a specified plane of motion; known as primary or prime movers, or muscles most involved.

Antagonist

Muscles that are usually located on the opposite side of the joint from the agonist and have the opposite action; known as contralateral muscles, they work in cooperation with agonist muscles by relaxing and allowing movement, but they perform the opposite motion of the agonist.

Stabilizers

Muscles that surround the joint or body part and contract to fixate or stabilize the area to enable another limb or body segment to exert force and move; known as fixators, they are essential in establishing a relatively firm base for the more distal joints to work from when carrying out movements.

Synergist

Muscles that aid or assist in the action of the agonists but are not primarily responsible for the action; known as guiding muscles, they assist in refined movement and rule out undesired motions. From a practical point of view, it is not essential that individuals know the exact force exerted by each of the elbow flexors—biceps, brachialis, and brachioradialis—in chinning. It is important to understand that this muscle group is the agonist or primary mover responsible for elbow joint flexion. Similarly, it is important to understand that these muscles contract concentrically when the chin is pulled up to the bar, and that they contract eccentrically when the body is lowered slowly. Antagonistic muscles are muscles that produce actions opposite those of the agonist. For example, the muscles that produce flexion of the elbow joint are antagonistic to the muscles that produce extension of the elbow joint. It is important to understand that specific exercises need to be given for the development of each antagonistic muscle group. The return movement to the hanging position at the elbow joint after chinning is elbow joint extension, but the triceps and anconeus are not being strengthened. A concentric contraction of the elbow joint flexors occurs followed by an eccentric contraction of the same muscles.

Fig. 6-1, *A* illustrates how the biceps is an agonist by contracting concentrically to flex the elbow. The triceps is an antagonist to elbow

FIG. 6-1 • Agonist-antagonist relationship. **A**, Biceps agonist in elbow flexion; **B**, triceps agonist in elbow extension.

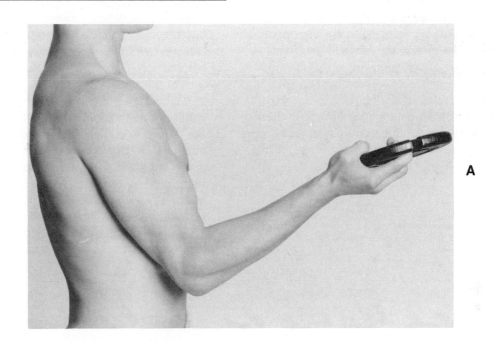

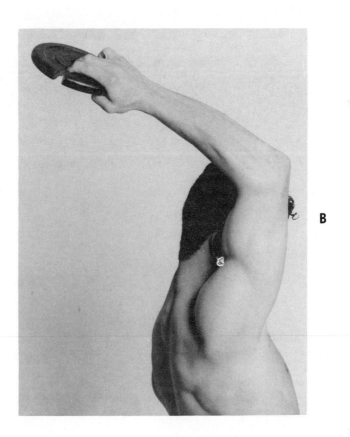

flexion, and the pronator teres is considered to be a synergist to the biceps in this example. If the biceps were to slowly lengthen and control elbow extension, it would still be the agonist, but it would be contracting eccentrically. Fig.6-1, *B* illustrates how the triceps is an agonist by contracting concentrically to extend the elbow. The biceps is an antagonist to elbow extension in this example. If the triceps were to slowly lengthen and control elbow flexion, it would still be the agonist, but it would be eccentically contracting. In both of these examples, the deltoid, trapezius, and various other shoulder muscles are serving as stabilizers of the shoulder area.

Upper extremity activities

Children seem to have an innate desire to climb, swing, and hang. Such movements use the muscles of the hands, wrists, elbows, and shoulder joints. But the opportunity to perform these types of activities is limited in our modern culture. Unless emphasis is placed on the development of this area of our bodies by physical education teachers in elementary schools, for both boys and girls, it will continue to be muscularly the weakest area of our bodies. Weakness in the upper extremities can impair skill development and performance in many common enjoyable recreational activities such as golf, tennis, softball, and raquetball. Athletes enjoy what they can do well, and they can be taught to enjoy activities that will increase the strength of this part of the body.

Chin-up (pull-up) FIG. 6-2

Description

The subject grasps a horizontal bar or ladder with the palms toward the face. From a hanging position on the bar, she pulls up until her chin is over the bar. Then she returns to the starting position.

Analysis

This exercise is separated into two movements for analysis: (1) movement upward to chinning position (concentric phase), and (2) return movement to hanging position (eccentric phase).

Movement upward to chinning position

Wrist and hand

Flexion

Wrist and hand flexors

Elbow joint

Flexion

Biceps brachii

Brachialis

Brachioradialis

Shoulder joint

Extension

Latissimus dorsi

Teres major

Posterior deltoid

Pectoralis major

Triceps brachii (long head)

Shoulder girdle

Adduction and depression

Trapezius (lower and middle)

Pectoralis minor

Rhomboids

Return movement to hanging position

Wrist and hand

Flexion

Wrist and hand flexors

Elbow joint

Extension

Elbow joint flexors (eccentric contraction)

Shoulder joint

Flexion

Shoulder joint extensors (eccentric contraction)

Shoulder girdle

Elevation and abduction

Trapezius (eccentric contraction)

Pectoralis minor (eccentric contraction)

Rhomboids (eccentric contraction)

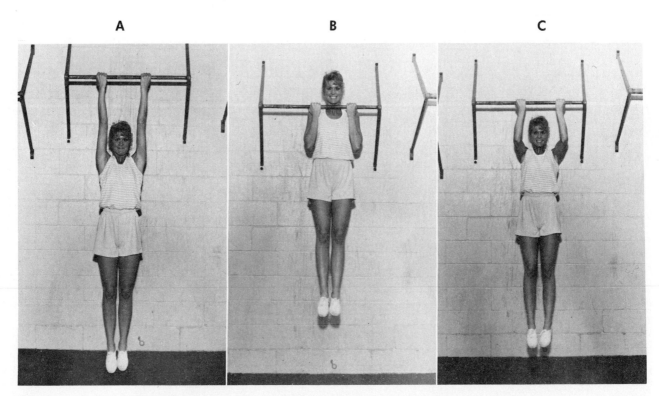

A   B   C

FIG. 6-2 • Pull-up. **A**, Straight-arm hang; **B**, chin over bar; **C**, bent-arm hang on way up or down.

Push-up (fingertip) FIG. 6-3

Description

The subject lies on the floor in a prone position with the legs together and the fingertips touching the floor with the hands pointed forward and approximately under the shoulders. Keeping the back and legs straight, the subject pushes up to a front-leaning rest position and returns to the starting position.

Analysis

This exercise is separated into two movements for analysis: (1) movement to front-leaning rest position (concentric phase), and (2) return movement to starting position (eccentric phase).

Movement upward to chinning position
Wrist and hand
Isometric contraction of wrist and hand flexors and extensors
Elbow joint
Extension
Triceps brachii
Anconeus
Shoulder joint
Flexion
Pectoralis major
Anterior deltoid
Biceps brachii
Coracobrachialis

Shoulder girdle
Abduction
Serratus anterior
Pectoralis minor

Return movement to starting position
Wrist and hand
Isometric contraction of wrist and hand flexors and extensors
Elbow joint
Flexion
Elbow joint extensors (eccentric contraction)
Shoulder joint
Extension
Shoulder joint flexors (eccentric contraction)
Shoulder gridle
Adduction
Shoulder girdle abductors (eccentric contraction)

Chins and push-ups are excellent exercises for the shoulder area, shoulder girdle, shoulder joint, elbow joint, and wrist and hand (see Fig. 6-3). Other exercises for this area are considered in Chapter 10. The use of free weights, Universal machines, and other conditioning exercises help develop strength and endurance for this part of the body.

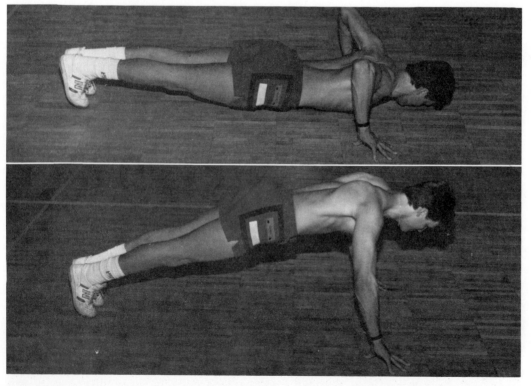

A

B

FIG. 6-3 • Push-up. **A**, Starting position; **B**, front-leaning rest position.

Latissimus pull (lats pull) FIG. 6-4

Description

From a sitting position the subject reaches up and grasps a horizontal bar (Fig. 6-4) at shoulder width apart. The bar is pulled down to a position behind the neck and shoulders. Then it is returned slowly to the starting position.

Analysis

This exercise is separated into two movements for analysis: (1) movement downward to a position behind the shoulders (concentric phase), and (2) return to the starting position (eccentric phase).

Movement upward to chinning position

Wrist and hand

Flexion

Wrist and hand flexors

Elbow joint

Flexion

Biceps brachii

Brachialis

Brachioradialis

Shoulder joint

Adduction

Pectoralis major

Anterior deltoid

Latissimus dorsi

Teres major

Subscapularis

Shoulder girdle

Adduction and depression

Trapezius (lower)

Rhomboid

Pectoralis minor

Return movement to starting position

Wrist and hand

Wrist and hand flexors

Elbow joint

Extension

Elbow joint flexors (eccentric contraction)

Shoulder joint

Abduction and elevation

Shoulder joint adductors (eccentric contraction)

Shoulder girdle

Abduction and elevation

Shoulder girdle adductors (eccentric contraction)

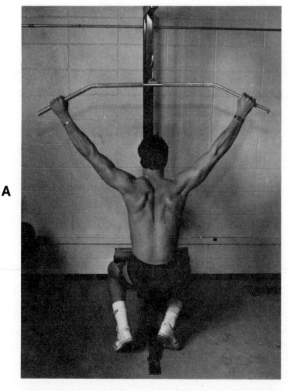 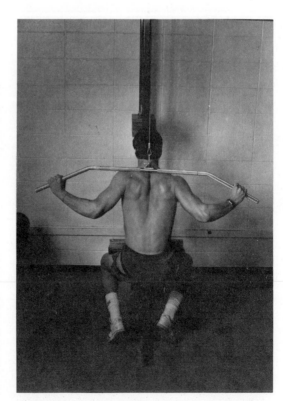

A
B

FIG. 6-4 • Latissimus pull (lats pull). **A,** Starting position; **B,** downward position.

Worksheet exercises

As an aid to learning, for in-class and out-of-class assignments, or for testing, a tearout worksheet is found at the end of the text (p. 222).

Dip exercise worksheet (no. 1)

List the movements that occur in each joint as the subject lowers himself in performing the dip and as he lifts himself. For each joint movement list the muscles primarily responsible and denote whether they are contracting concentrically or eccentrically.

Laboratory and review exercises

1. Analyze other conditioning exercises that involve the shoulder area.
2. Observe and analyze shoulder muscular activities of children on playground apparatus.
3. Discuss how you would teach boys and girls who cannot perform one chin-up to learn to do chin-ups. To do more push-ups.
4. Should boys and girls do chin-ups and push-ups to see whether they have adequate strength in this area of the body?
5. Test yourself doing chin-ups and push-ups to see whether you have adequate strength in this area of the body.
6. Why are push-ups better when done from the fingertips than with the hands flat on the floor?

References

Adrian M: Isokinetic exercise, Training and conditioning 1:1, June 1991.

Bouche J: Three essential lifts for high school players, Scholastic Coach 56:42, April 1987.

Brzycki M: R for a safe productive strength program, Scholastic Coach 57:70, September 1987.

Epley B: Getting elementary muscles, Coach and Athlete 44:60, November-December, 1981.

Matheson O, et al: Stress fractures in athletes, American Journal of Sports Medicine 15:46, January-February 1987.

Schlitz J: The athlete's daily dozen stretches, Athletic Journal 66:20, November 1985.

The hip joint and pelvic girdle

7

Objectives

• **To identify on a human skeleton or living subject the most important bone features of the hip joint and pelvic girdle.**

• **To label on a skeletal chart the most important bone features of the hip joint and pelvic girdle.**

• **To draw on a skeletal chart the individual muscles of the hip joint.**

• **To demonstrate with a fellow student all the movements of the hip joint and pelvic girdle.**

• **To palpate on a human subject the muscles of the hip joint and pelvic girdle.**

• **To list and organize the primary muscles that produce movement of the hip joint and pelvic girdle.**

Bones FIGS. 7-1 to 7-3

The hip joint is the ball and socket joint that consists of the head of the femur connecting with the acetabulum of the pelvic girdle. The pelvic girdle consists of a right and left pelvic bone joined together posteriorly by the sacrum. The femur is the longest bone in the body. The sacrum can be considered an extension of the spinal column with five fused vertebrae. The pelvic bones are made up of three bones: the ilium, the ischium, and the pubis. At birth and during growth and development they are three distinct bones. At maturity they are fused to form one pelvic bone.

The pelvic bone can be divided roughly into three areas from the acetabulum:
Upper two fifths = ilium
Posterior and lower two fifths = ischium
Anterior and lower one fifth = pubis

Joints FIGS. 7-1 to 7-3

In the anterior area, the pelvic bones are joined together to form the symphysis pubis, an amphiarthrodial joint. In the posterior area the sacrum is located between the two pelvic bones and forms the sacroiliac joints. Strong ligaments unite these bones and form rigid, immovable joints. The bones are large and heavy and for the most part are covered by thick, heavy muscles. Isolated joint movements can occur in this area. A good example is hip flexion when lying on one's back. However, movements usually involve the entire pelvic girdle and hip joints. In walking there is hip flexion and extension with rotation of the pelvic girdle, forward in hip flexion and backward in hip extension. Jogging and running result in faster and greater range of these movements.

Sport skills, such as kicking a football or soccer ball, are other good examples of hip and pelvic movements. Pelvic rotation helps increase the length of the stride in running; in kicking it results in a greater distance or more speed to the kick.

Except for the glenohumeral joint, the hip joint is one of the most mobile joints of the body, largely because of its multiaxial arrangement. Unlike the glenohumeral, the hip joints' bony architecture provides a great deal of stability, resulting in relatively few hip joint subluxations and dislocations. The hip joint is classified as an enarthrodial type joint and is formed by the

FIG. 7-1 • Right pelvic bone.

From Anthony CP, Kolthoff NJ: Textbook of anatomy and physiology, ed 9, St. Louis, 1975, Mosby.

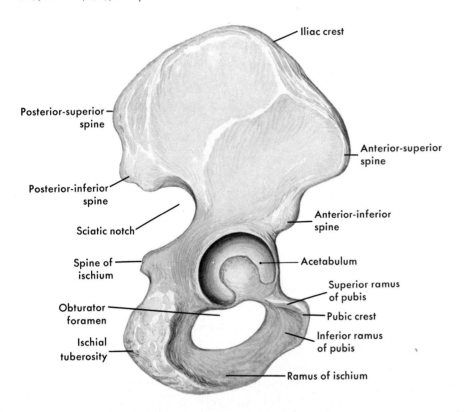

Iliac crest

Posterior-superior spine

Anterior-superior spine

Posterior-inferior spine

Sciatic notch

Anterior-inferior spine

Spine of ischium

Acetabulum

Superior ramus of pubis

Obturator foramen

Pubic crest

Inferior ramus of pubis

Ischial tuberosity

Ramus of ischium

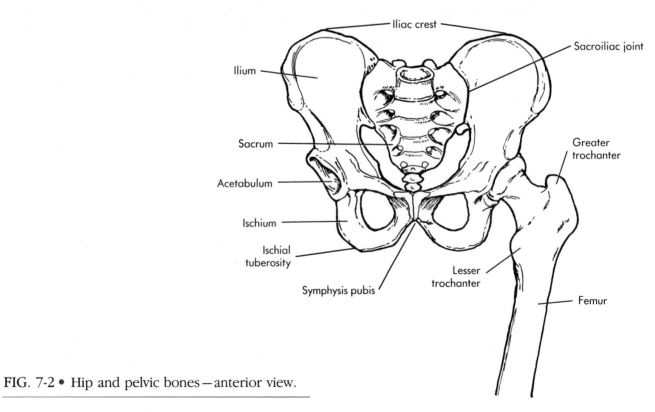

Iliac crest

Sacroiliac joint

Ilium

Sacrum

Greater trochanter

Acetabulum

Ischium

Ischial tuberosity

Lesser trochanter

Symphysis pubis

Femur

FIG. 7-2 • Hip and pelvic bones—anterior view.

TABLE 7-1 • Motions accompanying pelvic rotation

PELVIC ROTATIONS	LUMBAR SPINE MOTION	RIGHT HIP MOTION	LEFT HIP MOTION
Anterior rotation	Extension	Flexion	Flexion
Posterior rotation	Flexion	Extension	Extension
Right lateral rotation	Right lateral flexion	Adduction	Abduction
Left lateral rotation	Left lateral flexion	Abduction	Adduction
Right transverse rotation	Left lateral rotation	Internal rotation	External rotation
Left transverse rotation	Right lateral rotation	External rotation	Internal rotation

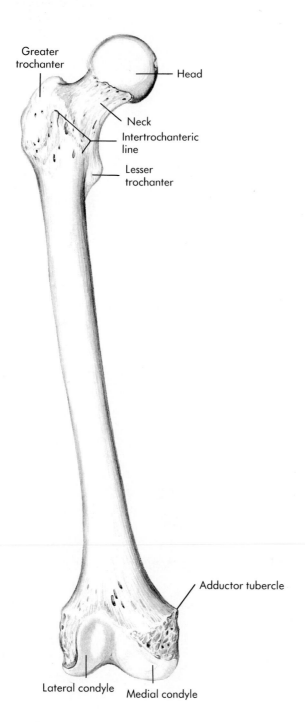

Greater trochanter

Head

Neck

Intertrochanteric line

Lesser trochanter

Adductor tubercle

Lateral condyle   Medial condyle

femoral head inserting into the socket provided by the acetabulum of the pelvis. An extremely strong and dense ligamentous capsule reinforces the joint, especially anteriorly.

Because of individual differences, there is some disagreement about the exact possible range of each movement in the hip joint, but the ranges are generally 0 to 130 degrees of flexion, 0 to 30 degrees of extension, 0 to 35 degrees of abduction, 0 to 30 degrees of adduction, 0 to 45 degrees of internal rotation, and 0 to 50 degrees of external rotation.

The pelvic girdle moves back and forth within three planes for a total of six different movements. To avoid confusion, it is important to analyze the pelvic girdle activity to determine the exact location of the movement. All pelvic girdle rotation actually results from motion at one or more of the following locations: the right hip, left hip, or the lumbar spine. Although it is not essential for movement to occur in all three of these areas, it must occur in at least one for the pelvis to rotate in any direction. Table 7-1 list the motions at the hips and lumbar spine that can often accompany rotation of the pelvic girdle.

FIG. 7-3 • Right femur, anterior surface.

From Anthony CP, Kolthoff NJ: Textbook of anatomy and physiology, ed 9, St. Louis, 1975, Mosby.

FIG. 7-4 • Movements of the hip with prime movers illustrated. **A,** Flexion; **B,** extension; **C,** adduction; **D,** abduction; **E,** internal rotation; **F,** external rotation.

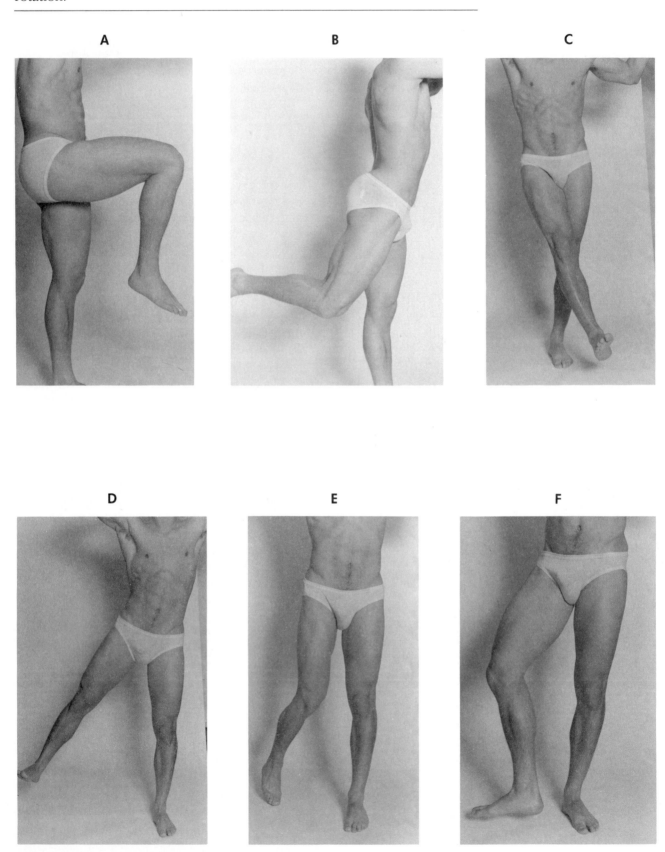

Movements FIGS. 7-4 and 7-5

Anterior and posterior pelvic rotation occur in the sagittal or anteroposterior plane, whereas right and left lateral rotation occur in the lateral or frontal plane. Right transverse (clockwise) rotation and left transverse (counterclockwise) rotation occur in the horizontal or transverse plane of motion.

Hip flexion: movement of the femur straight anteriorly toward the pelvis.

Hip extension: movement of the femur straight posteriorly away from the pelvis.

Hip abduction: movement of the femur laterally to the side away from the midline.

Hip adduction: movement of the femur medially toward the midline.

Hip external rotation: rotary movement of the femur laterally around its longitudinal axis away from the midline.

Hip internal rotation: rotary movement of the femur medially around its longitudinal axis toward to the midline.

Anterior pelvic rotation: anterior movement of the upper pelvis; the iliac crest tilts forward in a sagittal plane.

Posterior pelvic rotation: posterior movement of the upper pelvis; the iliac crest tilts backward in a sagittal plane.

Left lateral pelvic rotation: in the frontal plane the left pelvis moves superiorly in relation to the right pelvis; either the left pelvis rotates upward or the right pelvis rotates downward.

Right lateral pelvic rotation: in the frontal plane the right pelvis moves superiorly in relation to the left pelvis; either the right pelvis rotates upward or the left pelvis rotates downward.

Left transverse pelvic rotation: in a horizontal plane of motion the pelvis rotates to the body's left; the right iliac crest moves anteriorly in relation to left iliac crest, which moves posteriorly.

Right transverse pelvic rotation: in a horizontal plane of motion the pelvis rotates to the body's right; the left iliac crest moves anteriorly in relation to right iliac crest, which moves posteriorly.

A   B   C   D

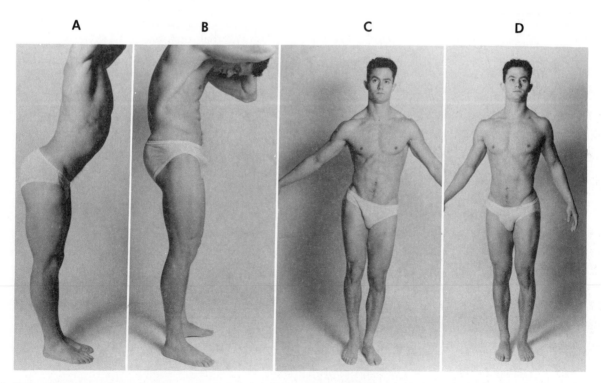

FIG. 7-5 • Pelvic girdle motions. **A**, Anterior pelvic rotation; **B**, posterior pelvic rotation; **C**, right lateral pelvic rotation; **D**, right transverse pelvic rotation.

Muscles

At the hip joint there are six two-joint muscles that have one action at the hip and another at the knee. The muscles actually involved in hip and pelvic girdle motions depend largely on the direction of the movement and the position of the body in relation to the earth and its gravitational forces. In addition, it should be noted that the body part that moves the most will be the part least stabilized. For example, when standing on both feet and contracting the hip flexors, the trunk and pelvis will rotate anteriorly; but when lying supine and contracting the hip flexors, the thighs will move forward into flexion on the stable pelvis.

In another example, the hip flexor muscles are used in moving the legs toward the trunk, but the extensor muscles are used eccentrically when the pelvis and the trunk move downward slowly on the femur and concentrically when the trunk is raised on the femur—this, of course, in rising to the standing position.

In the downward phase of the knee-bend exercise, the movement at hips and knees is flexion. The muscles involved primarily are the hip and knee extensors in eccentric contraction.

Hip joint and pelvic girdle muscles—location

Muscle location largely determines the muscle action. Sixteen or more muscles are found in the area (the six external rotators are counted as one muscle). Most hip joint and pelvic girdle muscles are large and strong.

Anterior
Primarily hip flexion
Iliopsoas
Pectineus
Rectus femoris*
Sartorius
Tensor fasciae latae
Medial
Primarily hip adduction
Adductor brevis
Adductor longus
Adductor magnus
Gracilis
Posterior
Primarily hip extension
Gluteus maximus
Biceps femoris*
Semitendinosus*
Semimembranosus*
External rotators
Lateral
Primarily hip abduction
Gluteus medius
Gluteus minimus
External rotators

---

*Two-joint muscles, knee actions are discussed in Chapter 8.

Iliopsoas muscle FIG. 7-6

(il′e-o-so′as)

Origin

Inner surface of the ilium, base of the sacrum, and sides of the bodies of the last thoracic (T12) and all the lumbar vertebrae (L1-5).

Insertion

Lesser trochanter of the femur and shaft just below.

Action

Flexion of the hip.
External rotation of the femur.

Palpation

Impossible to palpate, except with almost complete relation of the rectus abdominis muscle.

Innervation

Lumbar nerve and femoral nerve (L2-4).

FIG. 7-6 • Iliopsoas muscle. *O*, Origin; *I*, insertion.

Modified from Anthony CP, Kolthoff NJ: Textbook of anatomy and physiology, ed 9, St. Louis, 1975, Mosby.

Functional application and strengthening

The iliopsoas muscle is powerful in actions such as raising the legs from a supine position on the floor. Its origin in the lower back tends to move the lower back anteriorly or, in the supine position, pulls the lower back up as it raises the legs. For this reason, lower back problems are felt many times in this activity and bilateral six-inch leg raises are usually not recommended. The abdominals are the muscles that can be used to prevent this lower back strain by pulling up on the front of the pelvis and thus flattening the back. Leg raising is primarily hip flexion and not abdominal action. Backs may be injured by strenuous and prolonged leg-raising exercises. The iliopsoas contracts strongly, both concentrically and eccentrically, in sit-ups, particularly if the hip is not flexed. Some anatomy books list this muscle as two muscles: the iliacus and the psoas.

The iliopsoas may be exercised by supporting the arms on a dip bar or parallel bars and then flexing the hips to lift the legs. This may be done initially with the knees flexed in a tucked position to lessen the resistance. As the muscle becomes more developed, the knees may be straightened to add more resistance.

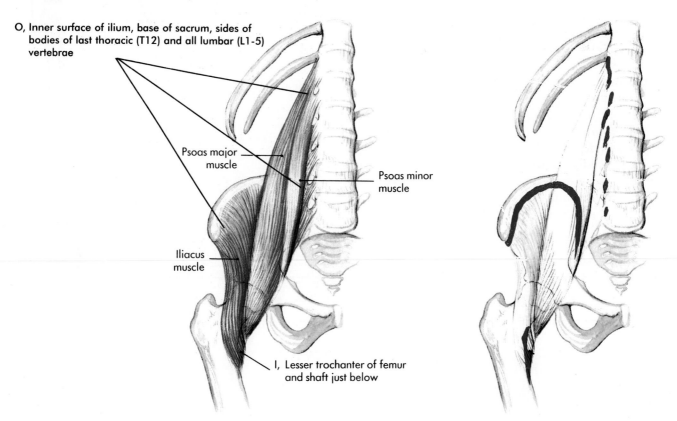

O, Inner surface of ilium, base of sacrum, sides of bodies of last thoracic (T12) and all lumbar (L1-5) vertebrae

Psoas major muscle

Psoas minor muscle

Iliacus muscle

I, Lesser trochanter of femur and shaft just below

Sartorius muscle FIG. 7-7

(sar-to′ri-us)

Origin

Anterior superior iliac spine and notch just below the spine.

Insertion

Anterior medial condyle of the tibia.

Action

Flexion of the hip.
Flexion of the knee.
External rotation of the thigh as it flexes the hip and knee.

Palpation

Easiest to palpate at the anterior superior spine of the ilium; impossible to palpate on subjects with medium and heavy legs.

Innervation

Femoral nerve (L2-3).

Functional application and strengthening

Pulling from the notch between the anterior superior and the anterior inferior spines of the ilium, the tendency again is to tilt the pelvis anteriorly (down in front) as this muscle contracts. The abdominal muscles must prevent this tendency by posteriorly rotating the pelvis (pulling up in front) and thus flattening the lower back.

The sartorius, a two-joint muscle, is effective as a hip flexor or as a knee flexor. It is weak when both actions take place at the same time. Observe that, in attempting to cross the knees when in a sitting position, one customarily leans well back, thus raising the origin to lengthen this muscle; making it more effective in flexing and crossing the knees. With the knees held extended, the sartorius becomes a more effective hip flexor. It is strengthened when hip flexion activities are performed as described for developing the iliopsoas.

FIG. 7-7 • Sartorius muscle. *O*, Origin; *I*, insertion.

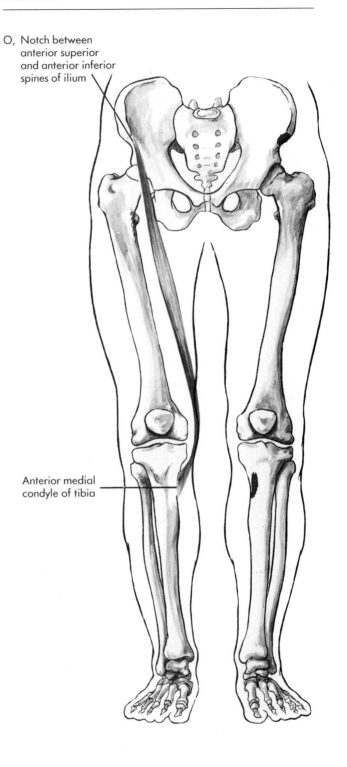

O, Notch between anterior superior and anterior inferior spines of ilium

Anterior medial condyle of tibia

Rectus femoris muscle FIG. 7-8

(rek'tus fem'or-is)

Origin

Anterior inferior iliac spine of the ilium.

Insertion

Superior aspect of the patella and patellar tendon to the tibial tuberosity.

Action

Flexion of the hip.
Extension of the knee.

Palpation

Any place on the anterior surface of the femur.

Innervation

Femoral nerve (L2-4).

Functional application and strengthening

Pulling from the anterior inferior iliac spine of the ilium, the rectus femoris muscle has the same tendency to anteriorly rotate the pelvis (down in front and up in back). Only the abdominal muscles can prevent this from occurring. In speaking of the hip flexor group in general, it may be said that many people permit the pelvis to be permanently tilted forward as they get older. The relaxed abdominal wall does not hold the pelvis up, and therefore an increased lumbar curve results.

A muscle's ability to exert force decreases as it shortens. This explains why the rectus femoris muscle is a powerful extensor of the knee when the hip is extended but is weak when the hip is flexed. This muscle is exercised, along with the vastus group, in running, jumping, hopping, and skipping. In these movements, the hips are extended powerfully by the gluteus maximus and the hamstring muscles, which counteract the tendency of the rectus femoris muscle to flex the hip while it extends the knee. It can be remembered as one of the quadriceps muscle group. The rectus femoris is developed by performing hip flexion exercises and/or knee extension exercises against manual resistance.

FIG. 7-8 • Rectus femoris muscle. *O,* Origin; *I,* insertion.

Modified from Anthony CP, Kolthoff NJ: Textbook of anatomy and physiology, ed 9, St. Louis, 1975, Mosby.

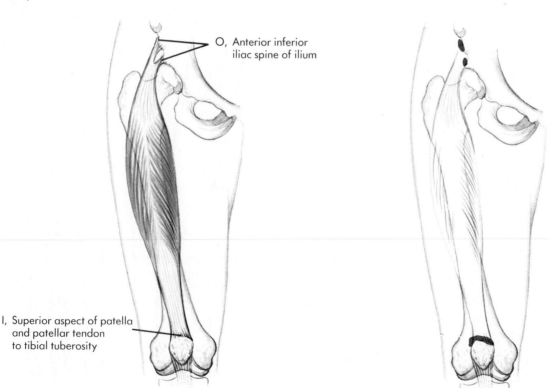

O, Anterior inferior
iliac spine of ilium

I, Superior aspect of patella
and patellar tendon
to tibial tuberosity

Tensor fasciae latae muscle FIG. 7-9

(ten'sor fas'i-e la'te)

Origin

Anterior iliac crest and surface of the ilium just below the crest.

Insertion

Iliotibial tract on the thigh one fourth of the way down.

Action

Abduction of the hip.
Flexion of the hip.
Tendency to rotate the hip internally as it flexes.

Palpation

Slightly in front of the greater trochanter.

Innervation

Superior gluteal nerve (L4-5, S1).

Functional application and strengthening

The tensor fasciae latae muscle aids in preventing external rotation of the femur as it is flexed by other flexor muscles.

The tensor fasciae latae muscle is used when flexion and internal rotation take place. This is a weak movement but important in helping to direct the leg forward so that the foot is placed straight forward in walking and running. Thus, from the supine position, raising the leg with definite internal rotation of the femur will call it into action.

The tensor fasciae latae may be developed by performing hip abduction exercises against gravity and resistance while in a sidelying position. This is done simply by abducting the hip that is up and then slowly lowering it back to rest against the other leg.

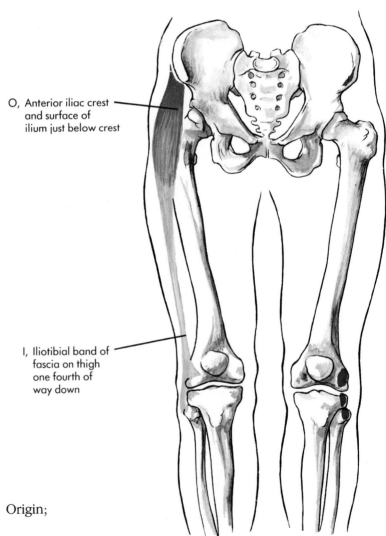

O, Anterior iliac crest and surface of ilium just below crest

I, Iliotibial band of fascia on thigh one fourth of way down

FIG. 7-9 • Tensor fasciae latae muscle. *O*, Origin; *I*, insertion.

Gluteus medius muscle FIG. 7-10

(glu′te-us me′di-us)

Origin

Outer surface of the ilium just below the crest.

Insertion

Posterior and middle surfaces of the greater trochanter of the femur.

Action

Abduction of the hip.
External rotation as the hip abducts (posterior fibers).
Internal rotation (anterior fibers).

Palpation

Slightly in front of and a few inches above the greater trochanter.

Innervation

Superior gluteal nerve (L4-5,S1).

Functional application and strengthening

Typical action of the gluteus medius and gluteus minimus muscles is seen in walking. As the weight of the body is suspended on one leg, these muscles prevent the opposite hip from sagging. Weakness in the gluteus medius and gluteus minimus can result in the Trendelenburg gait. With this weakness, the individual's opposite hip will sag upon weight bearing because the hip abductors can not maintain proper alignment.

Hip external rotation exercises performed against resistance can provide some strengthening for the gluteus medius, but it is best strengthened by performing the sidelying leg raises or hip abduction exercises as described for the tensor fascia latae.

FIG. 7-10 • Gluteus medius muscle. *O,* Origin; *I,* insertion.

Modified from Anthony CP, Kolthoff NJ: Textbook of anatomy and physiology, ed 9, St. Louis, 1975, Mosby.

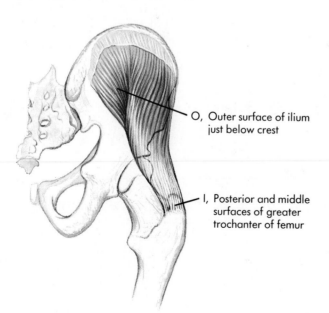

O, Outer surface of ilium just below crest

I, Posterior and middle surfaces of greater trochanter of femur

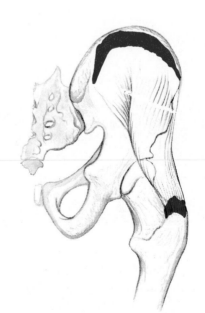

Gluteus minimus muscle FIG. 7-11

(glu'te-us min'i-mus)

Origin

Lateral surface of the ilium just below the origin of the gluteus medius.

Insertion

Anterior surface of the greater trochanter of the femur.

Action

Abduction of the hip.

Internal rotation as the femur abducts.

Palpation

Cannot be palpated.

Innervation

Superior gluteal nerve (L4-5, S1).

Functional application and strengthening

Both the gluteus minimus and medius are used powerfully maintaining proper hip abduction while running. As a result, both of these muscles are exercised effectively in running, hopping, and skipping, where weight is transferred forcefully from one foot to the other. As the body ages, the gluteus medius and gluteus minimus muscles tend to lose their effectiveness. The spring of youth, as far as the hips are concerned, resides in these muscles. To have great drive in the legs, these muscles must be fully developed.

The gluteus minimus is best strengthened by performing hip abduction exercises similar to the ones described for the tensor fascia latae and gluteus medius muscles. It may also be developed by performing hip internal rotation exercises against manual resistance.

FIG. 7-11 • Gluteus minimus muscle. *O,* Origin; *I,* insertion.

Modified from Anthony CP, Kolthoff NJ: Textbook of anatomy and physiology, ed 9, 1975, St. Louis, Mosby.

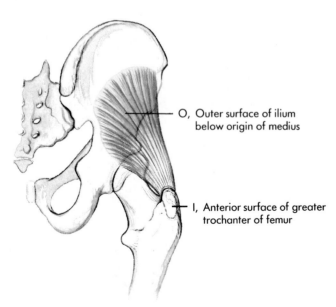

O, Outer surface of ilium below origin of medius

I, Anterior surface of greater trochanter of femur

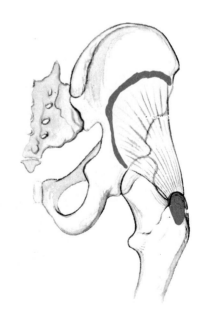

Gluteus maximus muscle FIG. 7-12

(glu′te-us maks′i-mus)

Origin

Posterior one fourth of the crest of the ilium, posterior surface of the sacrum near the ilium, and fascia of the lumbar area.

Insertion

Gluteal line of femur and iliotibial band of fascia latae.

Action

Extension of the hip.
External rotation of the hip.
Lower fibers, which assist in adduction.

Palpation

Wide area on the posterior surface of the pelvis.

Innervation

Inferior gluteal nerve (L5, S1-2).

Functional application and strengthening

The gluteus maximus muscle comes into action when movement between the pelvis and the femur approaches and goes beyond 15 degrees of extension. As a result, it is not used extensively in ordinary walking. It is important in extension of the thigh with external rotation.

Strong action of the gluteus maximus muscle is seen in running, hopping, skipping, and jumping. Powerful extension of the thigh is secured in the return to standing from a squatting position, especially if a barbell with weights is placed on the shoulders.

Hip extension exercises from a forward-leaning or prone position may be used to develop this muscle. This muscle is most emphasized when the hip starts from a flexed position and moves to full extension with the knee flexed 30 degrees or more to reduce the hamstrings involvement in the action.

FIG. 7-12 • Gluteus maximus muscle. *O,* Origin; *I,* insertion.

Modified from Anthony CP, Kolthoff NJ: Textbook of anatomy and physiology, ed 9, St. Louis, 1975, Mosby.

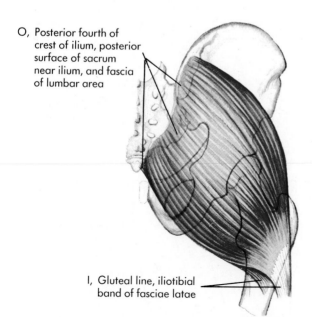

O, Posterior fourth of crest of ilium, posterior surface of sacrum near ilium, and fascia of lumbar area

I, Gluteal line, iliotibial band of fasciae latae

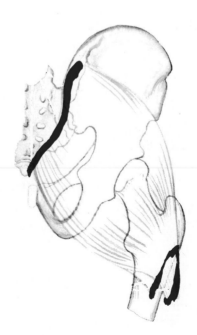

Six deep lateral rotator muscles—piriformis FIG. 7-13

(pi-ri-for′mis)

Gemellus superior

(je-mel′us su-pe′ri-or)

Gemellus inferior

(je-mel′us in-fe′ri-or)

Obturator externus

(ob-tu-ra′tor eks-ter′nus)

Obturator internus

(ob-tu-ra′tor in-ter′nus)

Quadratus femoris

(kwad-ra′tus fem′or-is)

Origin

Anterior sacrum, posterior portions of the ischium, and obturator foramen.

Insertion

Superior and posterior aspect of the greater trochanter.

Action

External rotation of the hip.

Palpation

Cannot be palpated.

Innervation

Piriformis: first or second sacral nerve (S1-2).
Gemellus superior: sacral nerve (L5, S1-2).
Gemellus inferior: branches from sacral plexus (L4-5, S1-2).
Obturator externus: obturator nerve (L3-4).
Obturator internus: branches from sacral plexus (L4-5, S1-2).
Quadratus femoris: branches from sacral plexus (L4-5, S1).

Functional application and strengthening

The six lateral rotators are used powerfully in movements of external rotation of the femur, as in sports in which the individual takes off on one leg from a preliminary internal rotation. Throwing a baseball and swinging a baseball bat, in which there is rotation of the hip, are typical examples.

Standing on one leg and forcefully turning the body away from that leg is accomplished by contraction of these muscles, and it may be repeated for strengthening purposes. A partner may provide resistance as development progresses.

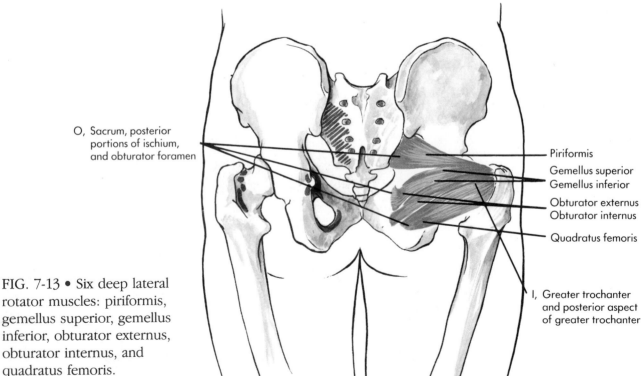

O, Sacrum, posterior portions of ischium, and obturator foramen

Piriformis
Gemellus superior
Gemellus inferior
Obturator externus
Obturator internus
Quadratus femoris

I, Greater trochanter and posterior aspect of greater trochanter

FIG. 7-13 • Six deep lateral rotator muscles: piriformis, gemellus superior, gemellus inferior, obturator externus, obturator internus, and quadratus femoris.

Biceps femoris muscle FIG. 7-14

(bi'seps fem'or-is)

Origin

Long head: ischial tuberosity.
Short head: lower half of the linea aspera, and lateral condyloid ridge.

Insertion

Head of the fibula and lateral condyle of the tibia.

Action

Extension of the hip.
Flexion of the knee.
External rotation of the hip.
External rotation of the knee.

Palpation

Lateral posterior side of the femur, near the knee.

Innervation

Long head: sciatic nerve—tibial division (S1-3).
Short head: sciatic nerve—peroneal division (L5, S1-2).

Functional application and strengthening

The semitendinosus, semimembranosus, and biceps femoris muscles are known as the hamstrings. These muscles, together with the gluteus maximus muscle, are used in extension of the thigh when the knees are straight or nearly so. Thus in running, jumping, skipping, and hopping these muscles are used together. The hamstrings are used without the aid of the gluteus maximus, however, when one is hanging from a bar by the knees. Similarly, the gluteus maximus is used without the aid of the hamstrings when the knees are bent while the hips are being extended. This occurs when rising from a knee-bend position to the standing position.

The biceps femoris is best developed through knee flexion exercises against resistance. Commonly known as hamstring curls or leg curls, they may be performed in a prone position on a knee table or standing with ankle weights attached. This muscle is emphasized when performing hamstring curls while attempting to maintain the knee joint in external rotation.

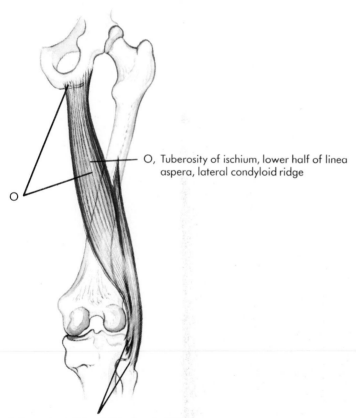

O, Tuberosity of ischium, lower half of linea aspera, lateral condyloid ridge

O

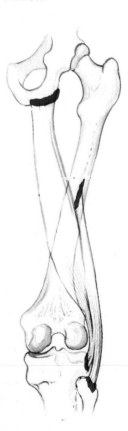

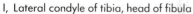

I, Lateral condyle of tibia, head of fibula

FIG. 7-14 • Biceps femoris muscle. *O,* Origin; *I,* insertion.

Modified from Anthony CP, Kolthoff NJ: Textbook of anatomy and physiology, ed 9, St. Louis, 1975, Mosby.

Semitendinosus muscle FIG. 7-15

(sem'i-ten-di-no'sus)

Origin

Ischial tuberosity.

Insertion

Upper anterior medial condyle of the tibia.

Action

Extension of the hip.
Flexion of the knee.
Internal rotation of the hip.
Internal rotation of the knee.

Palpation

Near the knee on the posteromedial side.

Innervation

Sciatic nerve—tibial division (L5, S1-2).

Functional application and strengthening

This two-joint muscle is most effective when contracting separately, either at the hip joint in extension or at the knee joint in flexion. When there is extension of the hip and flexion of the knee at the same time, both movements are weak. When the trunk is bent forward with the knees straight, the hamstring muscles have a powerful pull on the rear pelvis and tilt it down in back by full contraction. If the knees are flexed when this movement takes place, one can observe that the work is done chiefly by the gluteus maximus muscle.

On the other hand, when the muscles are used in powerful flexion of the knees, as in hanging by the knees from a bar, the flexors of the hip come into action to raise the origin of these muscles and make them more effective as knee flexors. By full extension of the hips in this movement, the knee flexion movement is weakened. These muscles are used in ordinary walking as extensors of the hip and allow the gluteus maximus to relax in the movement.

The semitendinosus is best developed through hamstring curls as described for the biceps femoris, but it is emphasized more if the knee is maintained in internal rotation throughout the range of motion.

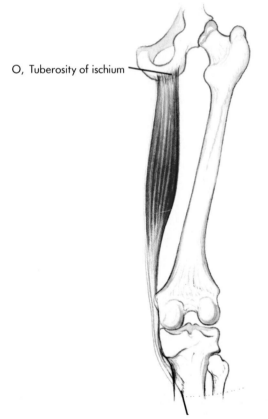

O, Tuberosity of ischium

I, Upper anterior medial condyle of tibia

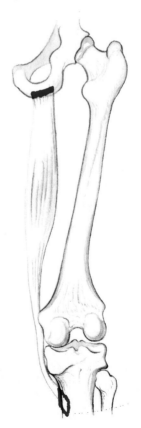

FIG. 7-15 • Semitendinosus muscle. *O,* Origin; *I,* insertion.

Modified from Anthony CP, Kolthoff NJ: Textbook of anatomy and physiology, ed 9, St. Louis, 1975, Mosby.

Semimembranosus muscle FIG. 7-16

(sem'i-mem'bra-no'sus)

Origin

Ischial tuberosity.

Insertion

Posterior surface medial condyle of the tibia.

Action

Extension of the hip.
Flexion of the knee.
Internal rotation of the hip.
Internal rotation of the knee.

Palpation

Largely covered by other muscles, the tendon can be felt at the posterior aspect of the tibia on the medial side.

Innervation

Sciatic nerve—tibial division (L5, S1-2).

Functional application and strengthening

Both the semitendinosus and semimembranosus are responsible for internal rotation of the knee, along with the popliteus muscle, which is discussed in the next chapter. Because of the manner in which they cross the joint, the muscles are very important to providing dynamic medial stability to the knee joint.

The semimembranosus is best developed by performing leg curls. Internal rotation of the knee throughout the range accentuates the activity of this muscle.

FIG. 7-16 • Semimembranosus muscle. *O,* Origin; *I,* insertion.

Modified from Anthony CP, Kolthoff NJ: Textbook of anatomy and physiology, ed 9, St. Louis, 1975, Mosby.

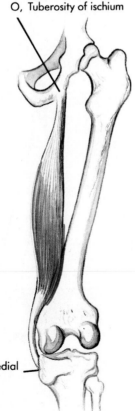
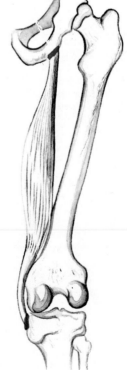

O, Tuberosity of ischium

I, Posterior surface medial condyle of tibia

Pectineus muscle FIG. 7-17

(pek-tin'e-us)

Origin

Space 1 inch wide on the front of the pubis just above the crest.

Insertion

Rough line leading from the lesser trochanter down to the linea aspera.

Action

Flexion of the hip.
Adduction of the hip.
Internal rotation of the hip.

Palpation

Angle between the pubic bone and the femur; hard to distinguish from the adductor longus muscle.

Innervation

Femoral nerve (L2-4).

Functional application and strengthening

As the pectineus contracts, it also tends to rotate the pelvis anteriorly. The abdominal muscles pulling up on the pelvis in front prevent this tilting action.

The pectineus muscle is exercised together with the iliopsoas muscle in leg raising and lowering. Hip flexion exercises, as well as hip adduction exercises, against resistance may be used for strengthening this muscle.

FIG. 7-17 • Pectineus muscle. *O,* Origin; *I,* insertion.

Modified from Anthony CP, Kolthoff NJ: Textbook of anatomy and physiology, ed 9, St. Louis, 1975, Mosby.

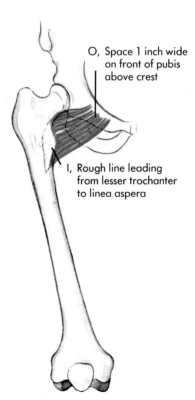

O, Space 1 inch wide on front of pubis above crest

I, Rough line leading from lesser trochanter to linea aspera

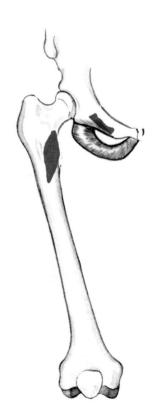

Adductor brevis muscle   Fig. 7-18

(ad-duk'tor bre'vis)

Origin

Front of the inferior pubic ramus just below the origin of the longus.

Insertion

Lesser trochanter and proximal one fourth of the linea aspera.

Action

Adduction of the hip.
External rotation as it adducts the hip.

Palpation

Cannot be palpated.

Innervation

Obturator nerve (L3-4).

Functional application and strengthening

The adductor brevis muscle, along with the other adductor muscles, provides powerful movement of the thighs toward each other. Squeezing the legs together toward each other against resistance is effective in strengthening the adductor brevis.

FIG. 7-18 • Adductor brevis muscle. *O*, Origin; *I*, insertion.

Modified from Anthony CP, Kolthoff NJ: Textbook of anatomy and physiology, ed 9, St. Louis, 1975, Mosby.

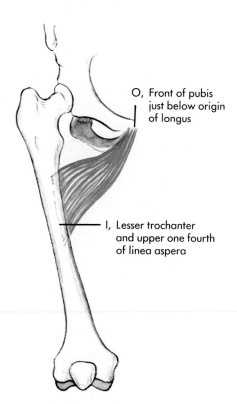

O, Front of pubis just below origin of longus

I, Lesser trochanter and upper one fourth of linea aspera

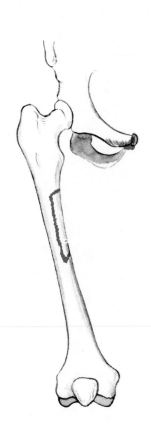

Adductor longus muscle FIG. 7-19

(ad-duk′tor long′gus)

Origin

Anterior pubis just below its crest.

Insertion

Middle third of the linea aspera.

Action

Adduction of the hip.
Assists in flexion of the hip.

Palpation

Just below the pubic bone on the medial side.

Innervation

Obturator nerve (L3-4).

Functional application and strengthening

The muscle may be strengthened by using the scissors exercise, which requires the subject to sit on the floor with the legs spread wide while the partner puts his legs or arms inside each lower leg to provide resistance. As the subject attempts to adduct his legs together, the partner provides manual resistance throughout the range of motion. This exercise may be used for either one or both legs.

FIG. 7-19 • Adductor longus muscle. *O,* Origin; *I,* insertion.

Modified from Anthony CP, Kolthoff NJ: Textbook of anatomy and physiology, ed 9, St. Louis, 1975, Mosby.

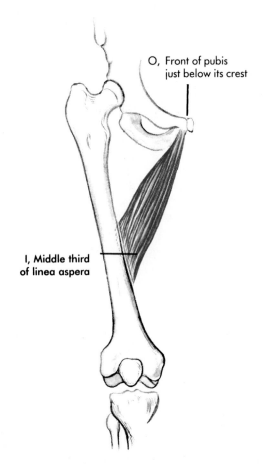

O, Front of pubis just below its crest

I, Middle third of linea aspera

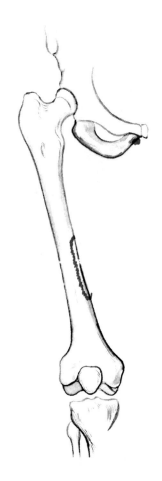

Adductor magnus muscle FIG. 7-20

(ad-duk'tor mag'nus)

Origin

Edge of the entire ramus of the pubis and the ischium and ischial tuberosity.

Insertion

Whole length of the linea aspera and adductor tubercle of medial femur.

Action

Adduction of the hip.
External rotation as the hip adducts.

Palpation

Posteromedial surface of the thigh.

Innervation

Anterior: obturator nerve (L2-4).
Posterior: sciatic nerve (L4-5, S1-3).

Functional application and strengthening

The adductor magnus muscle is used in the breaststroke kick in swimming or in horseback riding. Since the adductor muscles (adductor magnus, adductor longus, adductor brevis, and gracilis muscles) are not heavily used in ordinary movement, some prescribed activity for them should be provided. Some modern exercise equipment includes machines engineered to provide resistance for hip adduction movement. Hip adduction exercises such as those described for the adductor brevis and the adductor longus may be used for strengthening the adductor magnus as well.

FIG. 7-20 • Adductor magnus muscle. *O,* Origin; *I,* insertion.

Modified from Anthony CP, Kolthoff NJ: Textbook of anatomy and physiology, ed 9, St. Louis, 1975, Mosby.

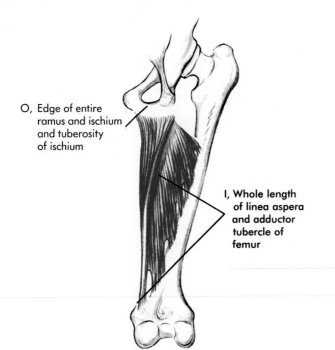

O, Edge of entire ramus and ischium and tuberosity of ischium

I, Whole length of linea aspera and adductor tubercle of femur

Gracilis muscle FIG. 7-21

(grasi'-lis)

Origin

Anteromedial edge of the descending ramus of the pubis.

Insertion

Anterior medial surface of tibia below the condyle.

Action

Adduction of the hip.
Flexion of the knee.
Internal rotation of the hip.

Palpation

Medial side of the thigh 2 to 3 inches below the pubic bone.

Innervation

Obturator nerve (L2-4).

Functional application and strengthening

The gracilis muscle performs the same function as the other adductors but adds some weak assistance to knee flexion.

The adductor muscles as a group (adductor magnus, adductor longus, adductor brevis, and gracilis) are called into action in horseback riding and in doing the breaststroke kick in swimming. Proper development of the adductor group prevents soreness after participation in these sports. The gracilis is strengthened with the same exercises as described for the other hip adductors.

FIG. 7-21 • Gracilis muscle. *O,* Origin; *I,* insertion.

Modified from Anthony CP, Kolthoff NJ: Textbook of anatomy and physiology, ed 9, St. Louis, 1975, Mosby.

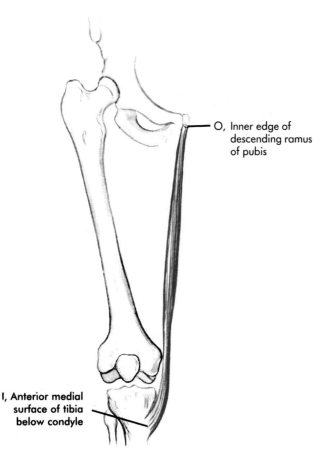

O, Inner edge of descending ramus of pubis

I, Anterior medial surface of tibia below condyle

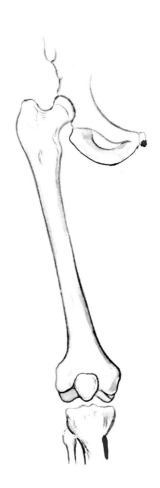

Muscle identification

In developing a thorough and practical knowledge of the muscular system, it is essential that individual muscles be understood. Figs. 7-22 and 7-23 illustrate groups of muscles that work together to produce joint movement.

FIG. 7-22 • Cross-section of left thigh at midsection.

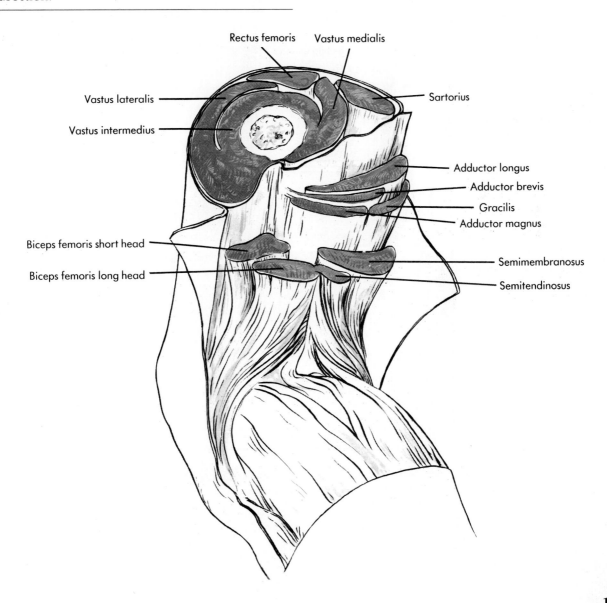

Modified from Anthony CP, Kolthoff NJ: Textbook of anatomy and physiology, ed 9, St. Louis, 1975, Mosby.

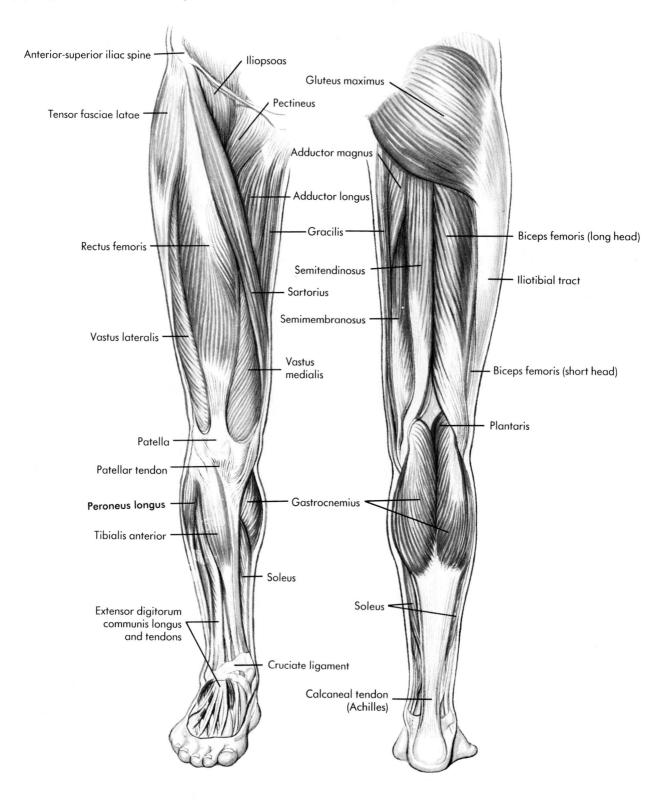

Anterior-superior iliac spine

Iliopsoas

Tensor fasciae latae

Pectineus

Gluteus maximus

Adductor magnus

Adductor longus

Gracilis

Rectus femoris

Biceps femoris (long head)

Semitendinosus

Sartorius

Iliotibial tract

Semimembranosus

Vastus lateralis

Vastus medialis

Biceps femoris (short head)

Patella

Plantaris

Patellar tendon

Peroneus longus

Gastrocnemius

Tibialis anterior

Soleus

Extensor digitorum communis longus and tendons

Soleus

Cruciate ligament

Calcaneal tendon (Achilles)

Worksheet exercises

As an aid to learning, for in-class and out-of-class assignments, or for testing, tearout worksheets are found at the end of the text (pp. 223 and 224).

Laboratory and review exercises

1. Locate the following parts of the pelvic girdle and hip joint on a human skeleton and on a subject.
   a. **Skeleton**
      (1) Ilium
      (2) Ischium
      (3) Pubis
      (4) Symphysis pubis
      (5) Acetabulum
      (6) Rami (ascending and descending)
      (7) Obturator foramen
      (8) Ischial tuberosity
      (9) Anterior superior iliac spine
      (10) Greater trochanter
      (11) Lesser trochanter
   b. **Subject**
      (1) Crest of ilium
      (2) Anterior superior iliac spine
      (3) Ischial tuberosity
      (4) Greater trochanter

2. How and where do you palpate the following muscles on a human subject?
   a. Gracilis
   b. Sartorius
   c. Gluteus maximus
   d. Gluteus medius
   e. Gluteus minimus
   f. Biceps femoris
   g. Rectus femoris
   h. Semimembranosus
   i. Semitendinosus
   j. Adductor magnus
   k. Adductor longus
   l. Adductor brevis

3. Be prepared to indicate on a human skeleton, using a long rubber band, where each muscle has its origin and insertion.

4. Distinguish between hip flexion and trunk flexion.

5. Demonstrate the movement and list the muscles primarily responsible for the following hip movements:
   a. Flexion
   b. Extension
   c. Adduction
   d. Abduction
   e. External rotation
   f. Internal rotation

6. How is walking different from running in relation to the use of the hip joint muscle actions?

7. The hip joint and pelvic girdle muscles are listed at the left of the chart on p. 116. Place a check in the column for each action of the muscle. Add a "P" for primary action.

Muscle analysis chart • Hip joint and pelvic girdle

Muscles	Flexion	Extension	Abduction	Adduction	External rotation	Internal rotation
Gluteus maximus						
Gluteus medius						
Gluteus minimus						
Biceps femoris						
Semimembranosus						
Semitendinosus						
Adductor magnus						
Adductor longus						
Adductor brevis						
Gracilis						
Lateral rotators						
Rectus femoris						
Sartorius						
Pectineus						
Iliopsoas						
Tensor fascia latae						

References

Daniels L, Worthingham C: Muscle testing: techniques of manual examination, ed 5, Philadelphia, 1986, Saunders.

Kendall HO, Kendall FP, Wadsworth GE: Muscles: testing and function, ed 2, Baltimore, 1971, Williams & Wilkins.

Lysholm J, Wikland J: Injuries in runners, American Journal of Sports Medicine 15:168, September-October, 1986.

Noahes TD, et al: Pelvic stress fractures in long distance runners, American Journal of Sports Medicine 13:120, March-April, 1985.

Perreira J: Treating the quadriceps contusion, Scholastic Coach 57:38, October 1987.

Sieg KW, Adams SP: Illustrated essentials of musculoskeletal anatomy, ed 2, Gainesville, Fl, 1985, Megabooks.

Stone RJ, Stone JA: Atlas of the skeletal muscles, Dubuque, Iowa, 1990, Brown.

The knee joint

8

Objectives

- To explain the cartilaginous and ligamentous structures of the knee joint.

- To draw and label on a skeletal chart muscles and ligaments of the knee joint.

- To palpate the superficial knee joint structures and muscles on a human subject.

- To demonstrate and palpate with a fellow student the movements of the knee joint.

- To name and explain the actions and importance of the quadriceps and hamstrings muscles.

- To list and organize the muscles that produce the movements of the knee joint.

The knee joint is the largest joint in the body and is very complex. It is primarily a hinge joint. The combined functions of weight bearing and locomotion place considerable stress and strain on the knee joint. Powerful knee joint extensor and flexor muscles, combined with a strong ligamentous structure, provide a strong functioning joint in most instances.

Bones

The enlarged femoral condyles articulate on the enlarged condyles of the tibia, somewhat in a horizontal line. Since the femur projects downward at an oblique angle toward, its medial condyle is slightly longer.

The top of the medial and lateral tibial condyles, known as the medial and lateral tibial plateaus, serve as a receptacle for the femoral condyles. The tibia is the medial bone in the leg bearing most of the weight of the lower leg. The fibula serves as the attachment for some very important knee joint structures, although it does not articulate with the femur or patella and is not part of the knee joint.

The patella is a sesmoid (floating) bone imbedded in the quadriceps muscle group and patella tendon. Its location helps provide a better angle of pull and thus a greater mechanical advantage for the quadriceps muscles in their work as knee extensors.

The knee joint is classified as a ginglymus joint because of its hingelike functioning into flexion and extension. However, it is sometimes referred to as a *trochoginglymus joint* because of the internal and external rotation movements that can occur during flexion.

The ligaments provide static stability to the knee joint, and contractions of the quadriceps and hamstrings produce dynamic stability. Cartilage forms the cushion between the bones (Fig. 8-1). The surfaces between the femur and tibia are protected by menisci (cartilages) attached to the tibia, which deepen the tibial fossa and act as a cushion between the bones.

The medial semilunar cartilage, or more technically, the medial meniscus, is located on the medial tibial plateau to form a receptacle for the medial femoral condyle; whereas the lateral semilunar cartilage (lateral meniscus) sits on the lateral tibial plateau to receive the lateral femoral condyle. Both of these menisci are thicker on their outside border and taper down very thin to the inside border. They can slip about slightly and are held in place by various small ligaments. The medial meniscus is the larger of the two and has a much more open C appearance than the rather closed C lateral meniscus configuration. One or both of the menisci may be torn in several different areas from a variety of mechanisms, resulting in varying degrees of severity and problems. These injuries often occur because of the significant compression and shear forces that develop as the knee rotates while flexing or extending during quick directional changes in running.

Two very important ligaments of the knee are the anterior and posterior cruciate, so named because they cross within the knee between the tibia and the femur. These ligaments are vital in respectively maintaining the anterior and posterior stability of the knee joint, as well as the rotatory stability (see Fig. 8-1).

The anterior cruciate ligament tear is one of the most common serious injuries to the knee. The mechanism for this injury is often one involving noncontact rotary forces associated with planting and cutting. Fortunately, the posterior cruciate ligament is not often injured. Injuries of the posterior cruciate usually come about through direct contact with an opponent or with the playing surface.

On the medial side of the knee is the medial (tibial) collateral ligament (see Fig. 8-1), which maintains medial stability by resisting valgus forces or preventing the knee joint from being abducted. Injuries to the tibial collateral occur quite commonly, particularly in contact or collision sports in which a teammate or opponent may fall against the lateral aspect of the knee or leg, causing medial opening of the knee joint and stress to the medial ligamentous structures.

On the fibular (outside) side of the knee, the fibular (lateral) collateral ligament joins the fibula and the femur. Injuries to this ligament are infrequent.

Other ligaments of lesser importance are located in the knee.*

The knee joint is well supplied with synovial fluid from a synovial cavity, which lies under the patella and between the surfaces of the tibia and the femur. Commonly, this synovial cavity is called the "capsule of the knee." More than 10 bursae are located in the knee, some of which are connected to the synovial cavity. Bursae are located where they can absorb shock or prevent friction.

The knee can usually extend to 180 degrees or a straight line, although it is not uncommon for some knees to hyperextend up to 10 degrees or more. When the knee is in full extension or 0 degrees of flexion, it can move from there to about 140 degrees of flexion. With the knee flexed 30 degrees or more, approximately 30 degrees of internal rotation and 45 degrees of external rotation can occur.

---

*More detailed discussion of the knee is found in anatomy texts and training manuals.

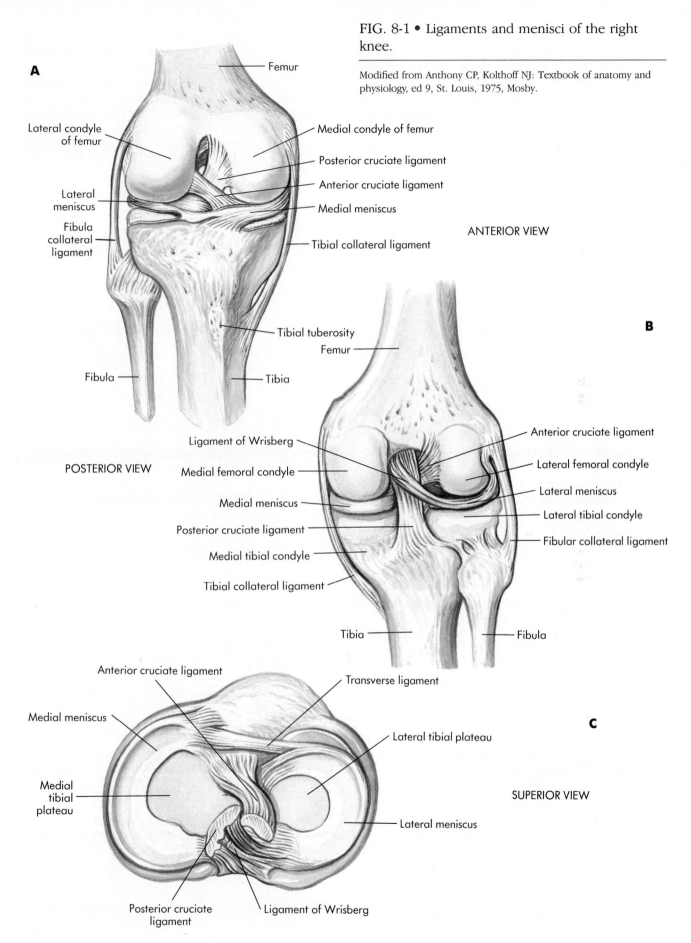

FIG. 8-1 • Ligaments and menisci of the right knee.

Modified from Anthony CP, Kolthoff NJ: Textbook of anatomy and physiology, ed 9, St. Louis, 1975, Mosby.

A

Femur

Lateral condyle of femur

Medial condyle of femur

Posterior cruciate ligament

Anterior cruciate ligament

Lateral meniscus

Medial meniscus

Fibula collateral ligament

Tibial collateral ligament

ANTERIOR VIEW

Tibial tuberosity

Fibula

Tibia

B

Ligament of Wrisberg

POSTERIOR VIEW

Medial femoral condyle

Medial meniscus

Posterior cruciate ligament

Medial tibial condyle

Tibial collateral ligament

Femur

Anterior cruciate ligament

Lateral femoral condyle

Lateral meniscus

Lateral tibial condyle

Fibular collateral ligament

Tibia

Fibula

Anterior cruciate ligament

Medial meniscus

Medial tibial plateau

Transverse ligament

Lateral tibial plateau

C

SUPERIOR VIEW

Lateral meniscus

Posterior cruciate ligament

Ligament of Wrisberg

Movements FIG. 8-2

Flexion and extension of the knee occur in the sagittal plane, whereas internal and external rotation occur in the horizontal plane.

Flexion: bending or increasing the angle of the knee characterized by the heel moving toward the buttocks.

Extension: straightening or increasing the angle between the femur and lower leg.

External rotation: rotary movement of the lower leg laterally away from the midline.

Internal rotation: rotary movement of the lower leg medially toward the midline.

FIG. 8-2 • Movements of the knee with prime movers illustrated. **A**, Extension; **B**, flexion; **C**, internal rotation; **D**, external rotation.

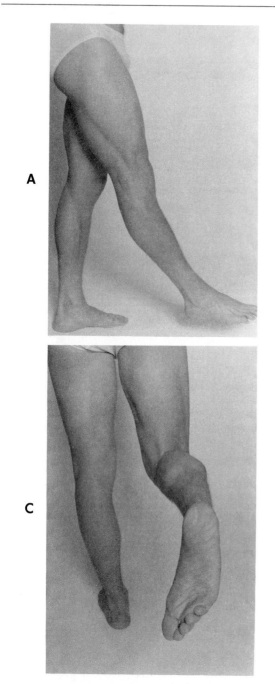

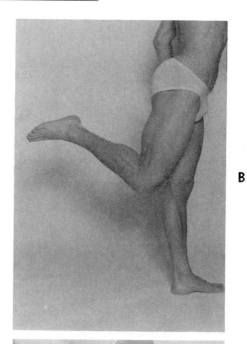

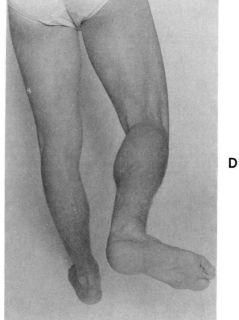

A

B

C

D

Muscles

Some of the muscles involved in knee joint movements were discussed in Chapter 7 because of their biarticular arrangement with both the hip and knee joints. As a result, they will not be covered again fully in this chapter. The knee joint muscles that have already been addressed are:

Knee extensor: rectus femoris.

Knee flexors: sartorius, biceps femoris, semitendinosus, semimembranosus, and gracilis.

The gastrocnemius muscle, discussed in Chapter 9, also assists minimally with knee flexion.

The muscle group that extends the knee is known as the quadriceps and consists of four muscles: the rectus femoris, the vastus lateralis, the vastus intermedialis, and the vastus medialis. The hamstring muscle group is responsible for knee flexion and consists of three muscles: the semitendinosus, the semimembranosus, and the biceps femoris. The semimembranosus and semitendinosus (medial hamstrings) muscles are assisted by the popliteus in internally rotating the knee, whereas the biceps femoris (lateral hamstring) is responsible for knee external rotation. Two-joint muscles are most effective when either origin or insertion is fixed by the contraction of the muscles that will prevent movement in the direction of the pull. All of the hamstring muscles, as well as the rectus femoris, are biarticular (two-joint) muscles.

As an example, the sartorius muscle becomes a better flexor at the knee when the pelvis is drawn up in front by the abdominal muscles, thus fixing the pelvis upward. This is exemplified by trying to flex the knee and cross the legs in the sitting position. One usually leans backward to flex the legs at the knees. Again, this is illustrated by kicking a football. The kicker invariably leans well backward to raise and fix the origin of the rectus femoris muscle to make it more effective as an extensor of the leg at the knee. Also, when youngsters hang by the knees, they flex the hips to fix or raise the origin of the hamstrings to make the latter more effective flexors of the knees.

Quadriceps muscles FIG. 8-3

(kwod'ri-seps)

The ability to jump is essential in nearly all sports. Individuals who have good jumping ability always have strong quadriceps muscles that extend the leg at the knee. The quadriceps functions as a decelerator when it is necessary to decrease speed to change direction. This deceleration function is also evident in stopping the body when coming down from a jump. The muscles are the rectus femoris (the only two-joint muscle of the group), vastus lateralis (the largest muscle of the group), vastus intermedius, and vastus medialis. All attach to the patella and by the patellar tendon to the tuberosity of the tibia. All are superficial and palpable except the vastus intermedius, which is under the rectus femoris. The vertical jump is a simple test that may be used to indicate the strength or power of the quadriceps. This muscle group is generally desired to be 25% to 33% stronger than the hamstring muscle group (knee flexors).

Rectus femoris muscle SEE FIG. 7-6

(rek'tus fem'o-ris)

Origin

Anterior inferior iliac spine.

Insertion

Superior aspect of the patella and patellar tendon to the tibial tuberosity.

Action

Flexion of the hip.
Extension of the knee.

Palpation

Any place on the anterior surface of the femur.

Innervation

Femoral nerve (L2-4).

Functional application and strengthening

When the hip is flexed, the rectus femoris becomes less effective as an extensor of the knee. The work is then done primarily by the three vasti muscles.

Also see rectus femoris, Chapter 7, p. 97, and above.

FIG. 8-3 • Quadriceps muscle group.

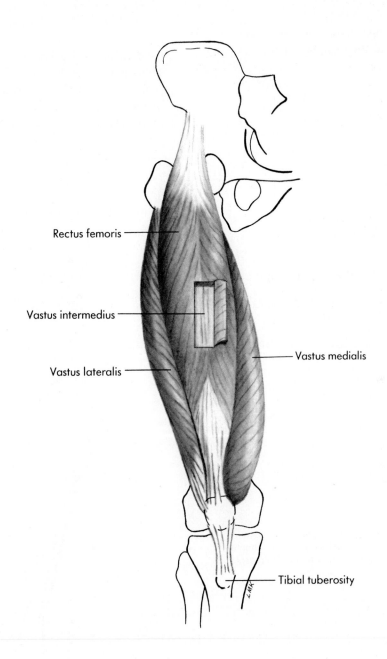

Rectus femoris

Vastus intermedius

Vastus lateralis

Vastus medialis

Tibial tuberosity

Vastus lateralis (externus) muscle

FIG. 8-4

(vas'tus lat-er-a'lis)

Origin

Lateral surface of the femur below the greater trochanter and upper half of the linea aspera.

Insertion

Lateral half of the upper border of the patella and patellar tendon to the tibial tuberosity.

Action

Extension of the knee.

Palpation

Anterior lateral aspect of the thigh.

Innervation

Femoral nerve (L2-4).

Functional application and strengthening

All three of the vasti muscles function with the rectus femoris in knee extension. They are used typically in walking and in running and must be used to keep the knees straight, as in standing. The vastus lateralis has a slightly superior lateral pull on the patella and, as a result, is occasionally blamed in part for common lateral patellar subluxation and dislocation problems.

FIG. 8-4 • Vastus lateralis muscle. *O,* Origin; *I,* insertion.

Modified from Anthony CP, Kolthoff NJ: Textbook of anatomy and physiology, ed 9, St. Louis, 1975, Mosby.

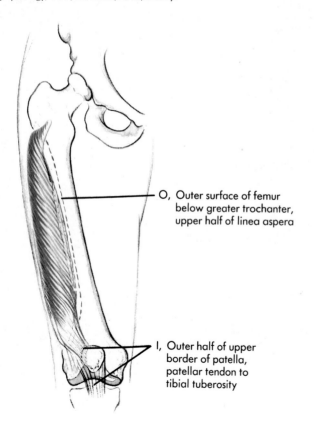

O, Outer surface of femur below greater trochanter, upper half of linea aspera

I, Outer half of upper border of patella, patellar tendon to tibial tuberosity

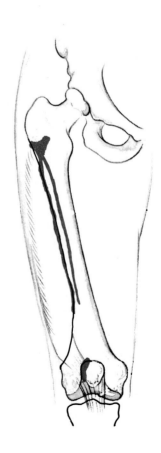

Vastus intermedius muscle FIG. 8-5

(vas'tus in'ter-me'di-us)

Origin

Upper two thirds of the anterior surface of the femur.

Insertion

Upper border of the patella and patellar tendon to the tibial tuberosity.

Action

Extension of the knee.

Palpation

Cannot be palpated; under the rectus femoris muscle.

Innervation

Femoral nerve (L2-4).

Functional application and strengthening

The three vasti muscles all contract in extension at the knee. They are used together with the rectus femoris in running, jumping, hopping, skipping, and walking. The vasti muscles are primarily responsible for extending the knee while the hip is flexed or being flexed. Thus, in doing a knee bend with the trunk bent forward at the hip, the vasti are exercised with little involvement of the rectus femoris. These natural activities mentioned develop the quadriceps.

Squats with a barbell of varying weights on the shoulders, depending on strength, are an excellent exercise for developing the quadriceps if done properly. Caution should be used, along with strict attention to proper technique to avoid injuries to the knees and lower back. Leg press exercises and knee extensions with weight machine apparatuses are other good exercises.

FIG. 8-5 • Vastus intermedius muscle. *O,* Origin; *I,* insertion.

Modified from Anthony CP, Kolthoff NJ: Textbook of anatomy and physiology, ed 9, St. Louis, 1975, Mosby.

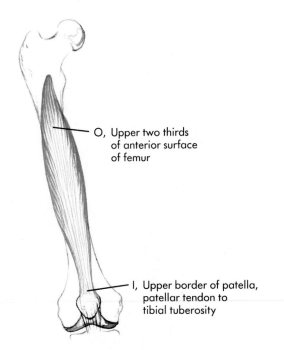

O, Upper two thirds of anterior surface of femur

I, Upper border of patella, patellar tendon to tibial tuberosity

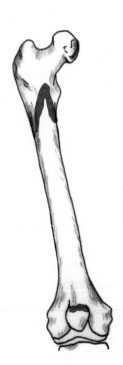

Vastus medialis (internus) muscle

FIG. 8-6

(vas'tus me-di-a'lis)

Origin

Whole length of the linea aspera and the medial condyloid ridge.

Insertion

Medial half of the upper border of the patella and patellar tendon to the tibial tuberosity.

Action

Extension of the knee.

Palpation

Anterior medial side of the thigh near the knee joint.

Innervation

Femoral nerve (L2-4).

Functional application and strengthening

The vastus medialis is thought to be very important in maintaining patellofemoral stability because of the oblique attachment of its distal fibers to the superior medial patella. This portion of the vastus medialis is referred to as the vastus medialis obliquus (VMO). The vastus medialis is strengthened similarly to the other quadriceps muscles by squats, knee extensions, and leg presses; but the VMO is not really emphasized until the last 10 to 20 degrees of knee extension.

FIG. 8-6 • Vastus medialis muscle. *O*, Origin; *I*, insertion.

Modified from Anthony CP, Kolthoff NJ: Textbook of anatomy and physiology, ed 9, St. Louis, 1975, Mosby.

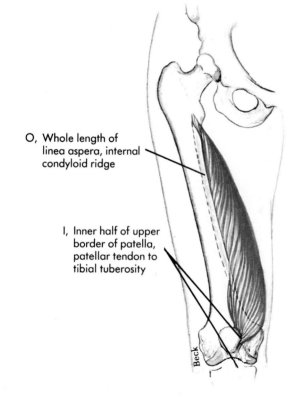

O, Whole length of linea aspera, internal condyloid ridge

I, Inner half of upper border of patella, patellar tendon to tibial tuberosity

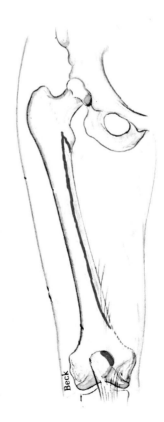

Hamstring muscles FIG. 8-7

Muscle strains involving the hamstrings are very common in football and other sports requiring explosive running. This muscle group is often referred to as the "running muscle" because of its function in acceleration. The hamstring muscles are antagonists to the quadriceps muscles at the knee and are named for their cordlike attachments at the knee. They include the biceps femoris, the semitendinosus, and the semimembranosus muscles. All of the hamstrings originate on the ischial tuberosity of the pelvic bone, and the semitendinosus and semimembranosus insert on the medial side of the tibia. The biceps femoris inserts on the lateral tibial condyle and head of the fibula — hence the saying, "Two to the inside and one to the outside." The second head of the biceps femoris is on the linea aspera of the femur.

Special exercises to improve the strength and flexibility of this muscle group are important factors in decreasing knee injuries. Inability to touch the floor with the fingers when the knees are straight is largely a result of a lack of flexibility of the hamstrings. The hamstrings may be strengthened by performing knee or hamstring curls on a knee table against resistance. The flexibility of these muscles may be improved by performing slow, static stretching exercises such as flexing the hip slowly while maintaining knee extension in a long sitting position.

The hamstrings are primarily knee flexors and secondarily hip extensors. Rotation of the knee can occur when it is in a flexed position. Knee rotation is brought about by the hamstring muscles. The biceps femoris externally rotates the lower leg at the knee. The semitendinosus and semimembranosus perform internal rotation. Rotation of the knee permits pivoting movements and change in direction of the body.

FIG. 8-7 • The hamstring muscle group.

From Arnheim DD: Modern principles of athletic training, ed 8, St. Louis, 1993, Mosby.

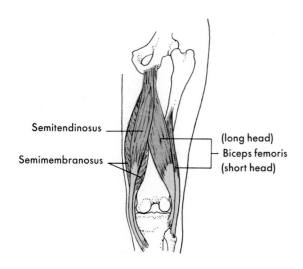

Popliteus muscle FIG. 8-8

(pop'li-te'us)

Origin

Posterior surface of the lateral condyle of the femur.

Insertion

Upper posterior medial surface of the tibia.

Action

Flexion of the knee.
Internal rotation of the knee.

Palpation

Cannot be palpated.

Innervation

Tibial nerve (L5, S1).

Functional application and strengthening

The popliteus muscle is the only typical flexor of the leg at the knee. All other flexors are two-joint muscles. It is vital to providing posterolateral stability to the knee. It assists the medial hamstrings in internal rotation of the lower leg at the knee.

Hanging from a bar with the legs flexed at the knee strenuously exercises the popliteus muscle. Also, the less strenuous activities of walking and running exercise this muscle. Specific efforts to strengthen this muscle combine knee internal rotation and flexion exercises against resistance.

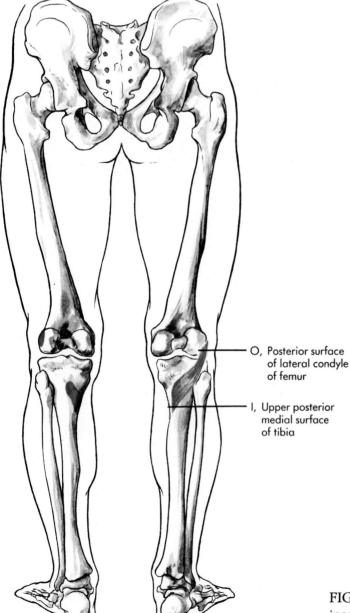

O, Posterior surface of lateral condyle of femur

I, Upper posterior medial surface of tibia

FIG. 8-8 • Popliteus muscle. *O,* Origin; *I,* insertion.

Worksheet exercises

As an aid to learning, for in-class and out-of-class assignments, or for testing, a tearout worksheet is found at the end of the text (pp. 225).

Posterior skeletal worksheet (no. 1)

Draw and label on the worksheet the knee joint muscles.

Laboratory and review exercises

1. Locate the following parts of bones on a human skeleton and on a subject:
   a. **Skeleton**
      (1) Head and neck of femur
      (2) Greater trochanter
      (3) Shaft of femur
      (4) Lesser trochanter
      (5) Linea aspera
      (6) Adductor tubercle
      (7) Medial femoral condyle
      (8) Lateral femoral condyle
      (9) Patella
   b. **Subject**
      (1) Greater trochanter
      (2) Adductor tubercle
      (3) Medial femoral condyle
      (4) Lateral femoral condyle
      (5) Patella

2. How and where do you palpate the following muscles on a human subject?
   NOTE: Palpate the previously studied hip joint muscles while they are performing actions at the knee.
   a. Gracilis
   b. Sartorius
   c. Biceps femoris
   d. Semitendinosus
   e. Semimembranosus
   f. Rectus femoris
   g. Vastus lateralis
   h. Vastus intermedius
   i. Vastus medialis
   j. Popliteus
3. Be prepared to indicate on a human skeleton, by a long rubber band, the origin and insertion of the muscles just listed.
4. Demonstrate the movements and list the muscles primarily responsible of the following movements:
   a. Extension of the leg at knee
   b. Flexion of the leg at knee
   c. Internal rotation of the leg at the knee
   d. External rotation of the leg at the knee
5. Discuss or have reports on the acceptability of deep knee-bends and duck-walk activities in a physical education program.
6. Prepare a report on the knee, including its ligamentous structure, joint structure, functioning, common injuries, and bracing for injuries.
7. Discuss or have reports on preventive and corrective exercises to strengthen the knee joint.
8. In the chart below list the muscles primarily responsible for knee joint movement.

Muscle analysis chart • Knee joint

Knee joint	
Flexion	Extension
Internal rotation	External rotation

References

Baker BE, et al: Review of meniscal injury and associated sports, American Journal of Sports Medicine 13:1, January-February 1985.

Evans W: Hamstring strength and flexibility development, Scholastic Coach 56:42, April 1987.

Garrick JG, Regna RK: Prophylactic knee bracing, American Journal of Sports Medicine 15:471, September-October 1987.

Kelly DW, et al: Patellar and quadriceps tendon ruptures — jumping knee, American Journal of Sports Medicine 12:375, September-October 1984.

Lysholm J, Wikland J: Injuries in runners, American Journal of Sports Medicine 15:168, September-October 1986.

Perreira J: Treating the quadriceps contusion, Scholastic Coach 57:38, October 1987.

Sieg KW, Adams SP: Illustrated essentials of musculoskeletal anatomy, ed 2, Gainesville, Fl, 1985, Megabooks.

Stone RJ, Stone JA: Atlas of the skeletal muscles, Dubuque, Iowa, 1990, Brown.

Wroble RR, et al: Pattern of knee injuries in wrestling, a six-year study, American Journal of Sports Medicine 14:55, January-February 1986.

The ankle and foot

9

. . . .

Objectives

• To identify on a human skeleton bones, ligaments, and arches of the ankle and foot.

• To draw and label on a skeletal chart the muscles of the ankle and foot.

• To demonstrate and palpate with a fellow student the movements of the ankle and foot.

• To palpate on a human subject the muscles of the ankle and foot.

• To list and organize the muscles that produce movement of the ankle and foot.

The complexity of the foot is evidenced by the 26 bones, 19 large muscles, many small (intrinsic) muscles, and more than 100 ligaments that make up the structure of the foot.

Support and propulsion are the two functions of the foot. Proper functioning and adequate development of the muscles of the foot and practice of proper foot mechanics are essential for everyone. In our modern society, foot trouble is one of the most common ailments. Poor foot mechanics begun early in life inevitably leads to foot discomfort in later years.

The fitness revolution that has occurred in the past two decades has resulted in great improvements in shoes available for sports and recreational activities. In the past, a pair of sneakers would suffice for most activities. Now there are basketball, baseball, football, jogging, soccer, tennis, walking, and cross-training shoes. Good shoes are important, but there is no substitute for adequate muscular development, strength, and proper foot mechanics.

Bones

Each foot has 26 bones that are shaped in the form of an arch. They connect with the upper body bony structure through the fibula and tibia (Figs. 9-1 and 9-2). Body weight is transferred from the tibia to the talus and the calcaneus.

In addition to the talus and calcaneus, there are five other bones in the rear foot known as the tarsals. Between the talus and the three cuneiform bones lies the navicular. The cuboid is located between the calcaneus and the fourth and fifth metatarsals. Anterior to the tarsals are the five metatarsals, which in turn correspond to each of five toes. The toes are known as the phalanges. There are three individual bones in each phalanx except for the great toe, which has only two. Each of these individual bones is known as a phalanx.

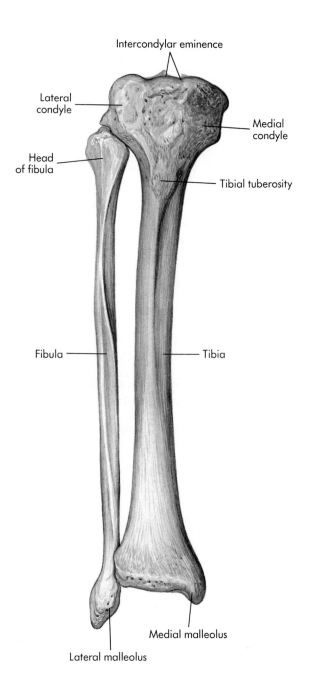

FIG. 9-1 • Right fibula and tibia.

From Anthony CP, Kolthoff NJ: Textbook of anatomy and physiology, ed 9, St. Louis, 1975, Mosby.

FIG. 9-2 • Right foot.

From Anthony CP, Kolthoff NJ: Textbook of anatomy and physiology,
ed 9, St. Louis, 1975, Mosby.

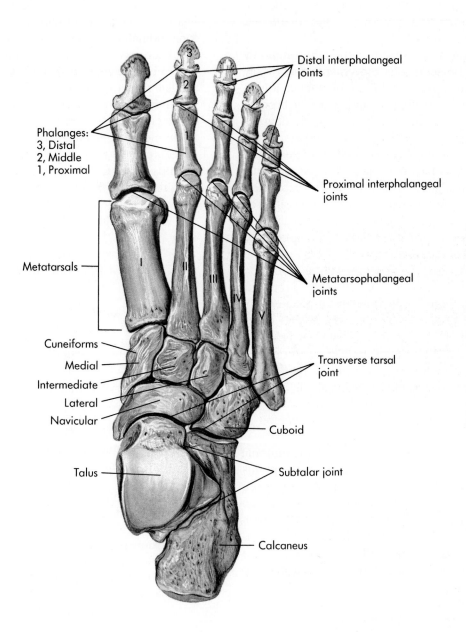

Phalanges:
3, Distal
2, Middle
1, Proximal

Distal interphalangeal
joints

Proximal interphalangeal
joints

Metatarsals

Metatarsophalangeal
joints

Cuneiforms

Medial

Intermediate

Lateral

Navicular

Transverse tarsal
joint

Cuboid

Talus

Subtalar joint

Calcaneus

Joints FIGS. 9-1 to 9-3

The ankle joint, technically known as the talocrural joint, is a hinge or ginglymus type joint. Specifically, it is the joint made up of the talus, the distal tibia, and the distal fibula. The ankle joint allows approximately 50 degrees of plantar flexion and 15 to 20 degrees of dorsiflexion. Greater range of dorsiflexion is possible when the knee is flexed, which reduces the tension of the biarticular gastrocnemius muscle.

Inversion and eversion, although commonly thought to be ankle joint movements, technically occur in the subtalar and transverse tarsal joints. These joints, classified as gliding or arthrodial, combine to allow approximately 20 to 30 degrees of inversion and 5 to 15 degrees of eversion. There is minimal movement within the remainder of the intertarsal and tarsometatarsal arthrodial joints.

The phalanges join the metatarsals to form the metatarsophalangeal joints, which are classified as condyloid-type joints. The metatarsophalangeal (MP) joint of the great toe flexes 45 degrees and extends 70 degrees, whereas the interphalangeal (IP) joint can flex from 0 degrees of full extension to 90 degrees of flexion. The MP joints of the four lesser toes allow approximately 40 degrees of flexion and 40 degrees of extension. The MP joints also abduct and adduct minimally. The proximal interphalangeal (PIP) joints in the lesser toes flex from 0 degrees of extension to 35 degrees of flexion. The distal interphalangeal (DIP) joint flexes 60 degrees and extends 30 degrees. There is much variation from joint to joint and person to person in all of these joints.

Ankle sprains are one of the most commonly occurring injuries in the physically active. Sprains involve stretching or tearing of one or more ligaments. There are far too many ligaments in the foot and ankle to discuss in this text, but a few of the ankle ligaments are shown in Fig. 9-3. Far and above the most common ankle sprain occurs as a result of excessive inversion that causes damage to the lateral ligamentous structures, primarily the anterior talofibular ligament and the calcaneofibular ligament. Excessive eversion forces causing injury to the deltoid ligament on the medial aspect of the ankle occur less commonly.

Ligaments in the foot and the ankle have the difficult task of maintaining the position of an arch. All 26 bones in the foot are connected with ligaments. This brief discussion is focused on the longitudinal and transverse arches.

There are two longitudinal arches (Fig. 9-4). The medial longitudinal arch is located on the medial side of the foot and extends from the calcaneus bone to the talus, the navicular, the three cuneiforms, and the proximal ends of the three medial metatarsals. The lateral longitudinal is located on the lateral side of the foot and extends from the calcaneus to the cuboid and proximal ends of the fourth and fifth metatarsals. Individual long arches vary from high, medium, and low, but a low arch is not necessarily a weak arch.

The transverse arch (see Fig. 9-4) extends across the foot from one metatarsal bone to the other.

Movements

Dorsiflexion: movement of the top of the ankle and foot toward the anterior tibia bone; accomplished by the extensor muscles of the ankle.

Plantar flexion: movement of the ankle and foot away from the tibia; accomplished by the flexor muscles of the ankle.

Eversion: turning the ankle and foot outward, away from the midline; weight on the medial edge of the foot.

Inversion: turning the ankle and foot inward, toward the midline; weight on the lateral edge of the foot.

Toe flexion: movement of the toes toward the plantar surface of the foot.

Toe extension: movement of the toes away from the plantar surface of the foot.

FIG. 9-3 • Right ankle joint. **A,** Lateral view; **B,** medial view.

From Seeley RR, Stephens TD, Tate P: Anatomy and physiology, ed 2, St. Louis, 1992, Mosby.

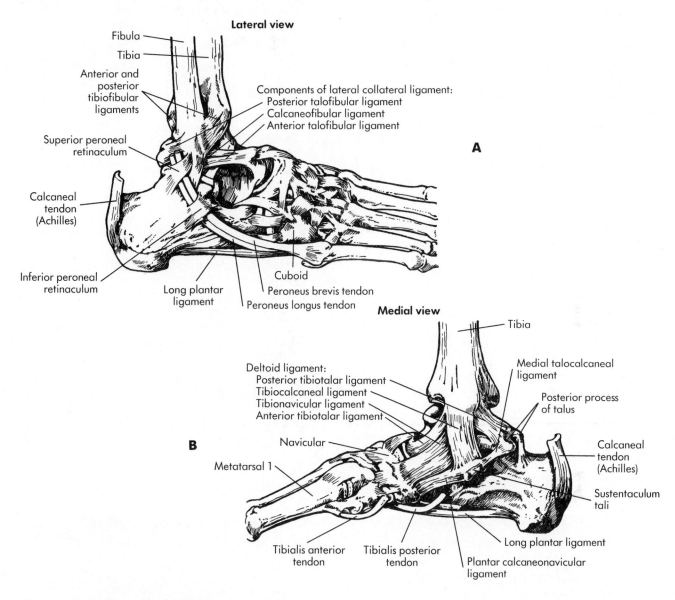

Lateral view

Fibula

Tibia

Anterior and posterior tibiofibular ligaments

Superior peroneal retinaculum

Calcaneal tendon (Achilles)

Inferior peroneal retinaculum

Components of lateral collateral ligament:
Posterior talofibular ligament
Calcaneofibular ligament
Anterior talofibular ligament

A

Cuboid
Peroneus brevis tendon
Peroneus longus tendon

Long plantar ligament

Medial view

Tibia

Deltoid ligament:
Posterior tibiotalar ligament
Tibiocalcaneal ligament
Tibionavicular ligament
Anterior tibiotalar ligament

Navicular

Metatarsal 1

B

Medial talocalcaneal ligament

Posterior process of talus

Calcaneal tendon (Achilles)

Sustentaculum tali

Long plantar ligament

Plantar calcaneonavicular ligament

Tibialis anterior tendon

Tibialis posterior tendon

FIG. 9-4 • Longitudinal and transverse arches.

From Anthony CP, Kolthoff NJ: Textbook of anatomy and physiology, ed 9, St. Louis, 1975, Mosby.

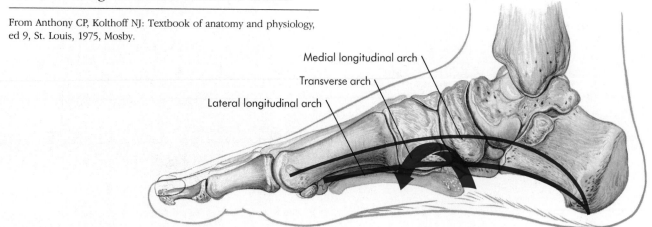

Medial longitudinal arch

Transverse arch

Lateral longitudinal arch

Ankle and foot muscles FIG. 9-5

The large number of muscles in the ankle and foot may be easier to learn if grouped according to location and function. In general, the muscles located on the anterior of the ankle and foot are the dorsal flexors. Those to the posterior are plantar flexors. Muscles that are evertors are located more to the lateral side, whereas the invertors are located medially.

NOTE: A number of the ankle and foot muscles are capable of helping produce more than one movement.

Plantar flexors
  Gastrocnemius
  Flexor digitorum longus
  Flexor hallucis longus
  Peroneus longus
  Peroneus brevis
  Plantaris
  Soleus
  Tibialis posterior
Evertors
  Peroneus longus
  Peroneus brevis
  Peroneus tertius
  Extensor digitorum longus
Dorsiflexors
  Tibialis anterior
  Peroneus tertius
  Extensor digitorum longus (extensor of lesser toes)
  Extensor hallucis longus (greater toe extensor)
Invertors
  Tibialis anterior
  Tibialis posterior
  Flexor digitorum longus (flexor of lesser toes)
  Flexor hallucis longus (great toe flexor)

FIG. 9-5 • Movements of the ankle and foot. **A**, Ankle dorsiflexion; **B**, ankle plantar flexion.

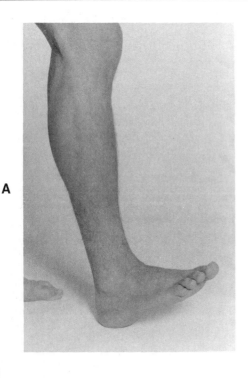
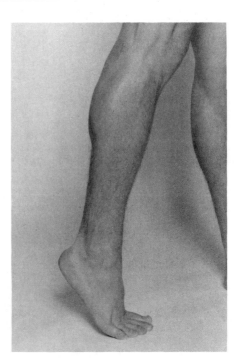

A

B

FIG. 9-5 cont'd • Movements of the ankle and foot. **C**, transverse tarsal and subtalar eversion; **D**, transverse tarsal and subtalar inversion; **E**, flexion of the toes; **F**, extension of the toes.

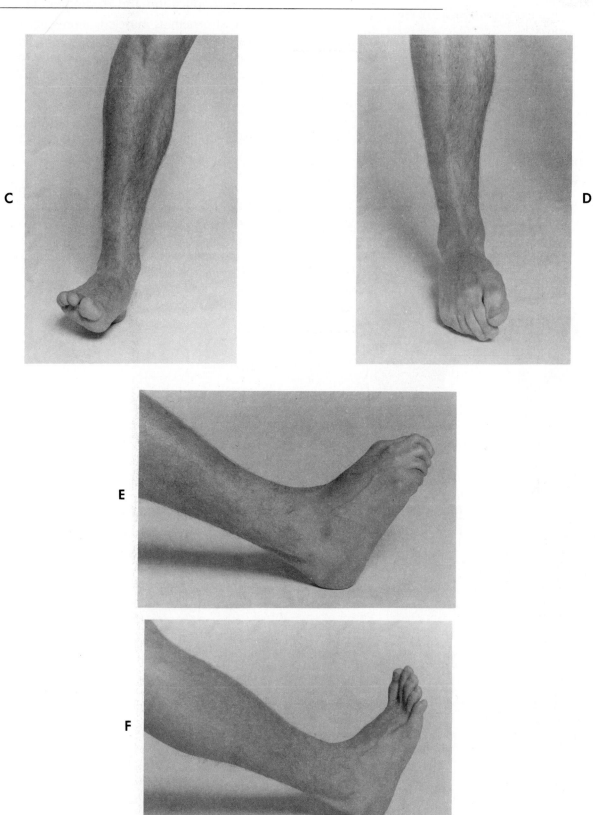

Gastrocnemius muscle FIG. 9-6

(gas-trok-ne'mi-us)

Origin

Medial head: posterior surface of the medial femoral condyle.
Lateral head: posterior surface of the lateral femoral condyle.

Insertion

Posterior surface of the calcaneus (Achilles tendon).

Action

Plantar flexion of the ankle.
Flexion of the knee.

Palpation

Easiest muscle in the lower extremity to palpate; upper posterior aspect of the lower leg.

Innervation

Tibial nerve (S1,S2).

Functional application and strengthening

The gastrocnemius muscle is more effective as a knee flexor if the foot is elevated and more effective as a plantar flexor of the foot if the knee is held in extension. This is observed when one sits too close to the wheel in driving a car. When the knees are bent, the muscle becomes an ineffective plantar flexor, and it is more difficult to depress the brakes. Running, jumping, hopping, and skipping exercises all depend significantly on the gastrocnemius and soleus to propel the body upward and forward. Heel-raising exercises with the knees in full extension and the toes resting on a block of wood are an excellent way to strengthen the muscle through the full range of motion. By holding a barbell on the shoulders, the resistance may be increased.

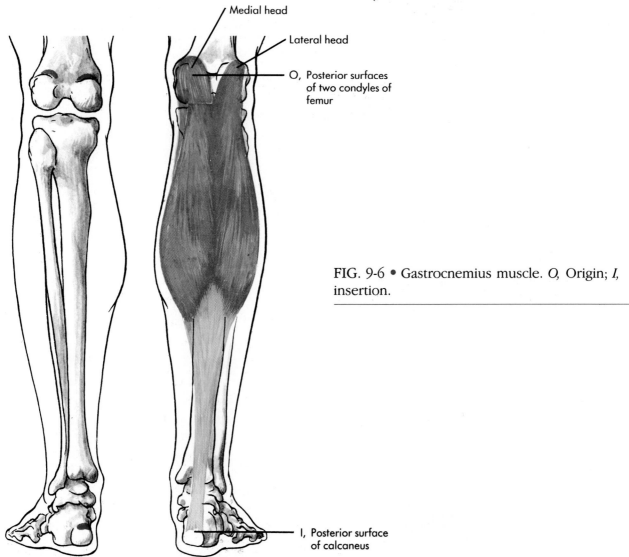

FIG. 9-6 • Gastrocnemius muscle. *O,* Origin; *I,* insertion.

Soleus muscles FIG. 9-7

(so'le-us)

Origin

Upper two thirds of the posterior surfaces of the tibia and fibula.

Insertion

Posterior surface of the calcaneus (Achilles tendon).

Action

Plantar flexion of the ankle.

Palpation

Under the gastrocnemius muscle on the lateral side of the lower leg.

Innervation

Tibial nerve (S1,S2).

Functional application and strengthening

The soleus muscle is one of the most important plantar flexors of the ankle. Some anatomists believe that it is nearly as important in this movement as the gastrocnemius. This is especially true when the knee is flexed. When an individual rises up on his toes, the soleus muscle can plainly be seen on the outside of the lower leg if one has exercised the legs extensively as in running and walking.

The soleus muscle is used whenever the ankle plantar flexes. Any movement with body weight on the foot with the knee flexed or extended calls it into action. When the knee is flexed slightly, the effect of the gastrocnemius is reduced, thereby placing more work on the soleus. Running, jumping, hopping, skipping, and dancing on the toes are all exercises that depend heavily on the soleus. It may be strengthened through any plantar flexion exercise against resistance, particularly if the knee is flexed slightly to deemphasize the gastrocnemius. Heel-raising exercises as described for the gastrocnemius, except with the knees flexed slightly, are one way to isolate this muscle for strengthening. Resistance may be increased by holding a barbell on the shoulders.

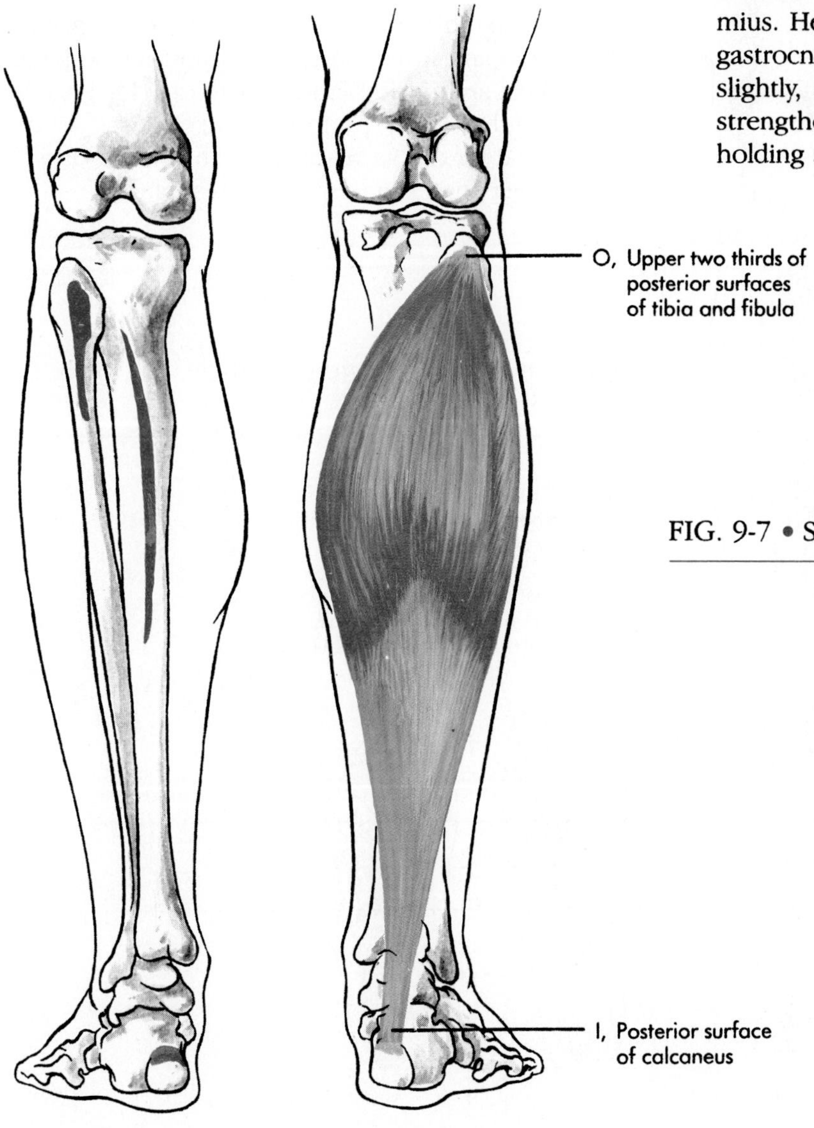

O, Upper two thirds of posterior surfaces of tibia and fibula

I, Posterior surface of calcaneus

FIG. 9-7 • Soleus muscle. *O,* Origin; *I,* insertion.

Tibialis posterior muscle FIG. 9-8

(tib-i-a′lis pos-te′ri-or)

Origin

Posterior surface of the upper half of the interosseus membrane and adjacent surfaces of the tibia and fibula.

Insertion

Lower inner surfaces of the navicular and cuneiform bones and bases of the second, third, fourth, and fifth metatarsal bones.

Action

Plantar flexion of the ankle.
Inversion of the foot.

Palpation

Cannot be palpated.

Innervation

Tibial nerve (L5, S1).

Functional application and strengthening

Passing down the back of the leg, under the medial malleolus, then forward to the navicular and medial cuneiform bones, the tibialis posterior muscle pulls down from the underside and contracts to invert and plantar flex the foot. "Shin splint" is a slang term frequently used to describe an often chronic condition in which the tibialis posterior, tibialis anterior, and extensor digitorum longus muscles may be inflammed. This inflammation is usually a tendonitis of one or more of these structures, but may be a result of stress fracture, periostitis, tibial stress syndrome, or a compartment syndrome. Sprints and long-distance running are common causes, particularly if the athlete has not developed appropriate strength, flexibilty, and endurance in the lower leg musculature.

Use of the tibialis posterior muscle in plantar flexion and inversion gives support to the longitudinal arch of the foot. This muscle is generally strengthened by performing heel raises as described for the gastrocnemius and soleus, as well as inversion exercises against resistance.

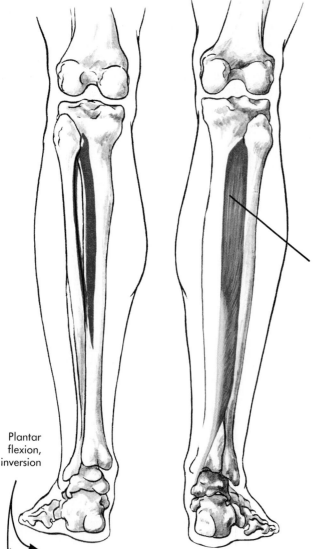

Plantar flexion, inversion

FIG. 9-8 • Tibialis posterior muscle. *O,* Origin; *I,* insertion.

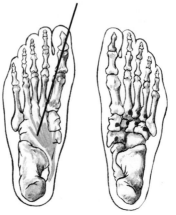

O, Posterior surface of upper half of interosseous membrane, adjacent surfaces of tibia and fibula

I, Lower inner surfaces of navicular and cuneiform bones, bases of second, third, fourth, and fifth metatarsal bones

Flexor digitorum longus muscle

FIG. 9-9

(fleks′or dij-i-to′rum long′gus)

Origin

Lower two thirds of the posterior surface of the tibia.

Insertion

Base of the distal phalanx of each of the four lesser toes.

Action

Plantar flexion of the four lesser toes.
Plantar flexion of the ankle.
Inversion of the foot.

Palpation

Cannot be palpated.

Innervation

Tibial nerve (L5,S1).

Functional application and strengthening

Passing down the back of the lower leg under the medial malleolus and then forward, the flexor digitorum longus muscle draws the four lesser toes down into flexion toward the heel as it plantar flexes the ankle. It is very important in helping other foot muscles maintain the longitudinal arch. Walking, running, and jumping do not necessarily call the flexor digitorum longus muscle into action. Some of the weak foot and ankle conditions result from ineffective use of the flexor digitorum longus. Walking barefoot with the toes curled downward toward the heels and with the foot inverted will exercise this muscle. It may be strengthened by performing towel grabs against resistance in which the heel rests on the floor while the toes extend to grab a flat towel and then flex to pull the towel under the foot. This may be repeated numerous times with a small weight placed on the opposite end of the towel for added resistance.

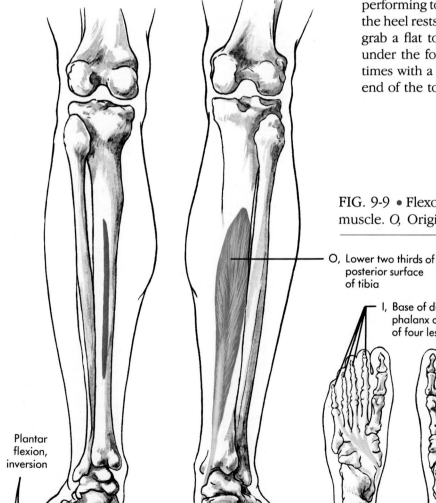

FIG. 9-9 • Flexor digitorum longus muscle. *O,* Origin; *I,* insertion.

O, Lower two thirds of posterior surface of tibia

I, Base of distal phalanx of each of four lesser toes

Plantar flexion, inversion

Flexor hallucis longus muscle FIG. 9-10

(fleks'or hal-u'sis long'gus)

Origin

Lower two thirds of the posterior surface of the fibula.

Insertion

Base of the distal phalanx of the big toe, under surface.

Action

Plantar flexion of the big toe.
Inversion of the foot.
Plantar flexion of the ankle.

Palpation

Anteromedial to the Achilles tendon near the heel.

Innervation

Tibial nerve (L5,S1,S2).

Functional application and strengthening

Pulling from the underside of the great toe, the flexor hallucis longus muscle may work independently of the flexor digitorum longus muscle or with it. If these two muscles are poorly developed, they cramp easily when they are called on to do activities to which they are unaccustomed.

These muscles are used effectively in walking if the toes are used (as they should be) in maintaining balance as each step is taken. Walking "with" the toes rather than "over" them is an important action for them.

When the gastrocnemius, soleus, tibialis posterior, peroneus longus, peroneus brevis, flexor digitorum longus, flexor digitorum brevis, and flexor hallucis longus muscles are all used effectively in walking, the strength of the ankle is evident. If an ankle and a foot are weak, in most cases it is because of lack of use of all the muscles just mentioned. Running, walking, jumping, hopping, and skipping provide exercise for this muscle group. The flexor hallucis longus muscle may be specifically strengthened by performing towel grabs as described for the flexor digitorum longus.

FIG. 9-10 • Flexor hallucis longus muscle. *O,*
Origin; *I,* insertion.

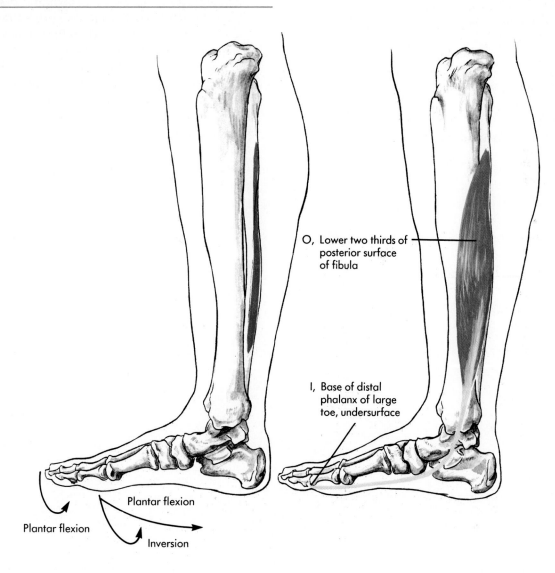

O, Lower two thirds of
posterior surface
of fibula

I, Base of distal
phalanx of large
toe, undersurface

Plantar flexion

Plantar flexion

Inversion

Peroneus longus muscle FIG. 9-11

(per-o-ne'us long'gus)

Origin

Head and upper two thirds of the lateral surface of the fibula.

Insertion

Undersurfaces of the medial cuneiform and first metatarsal bones.

Action

Eversion of the foot.
Plantar flexion of the ankle.

Palpation

Third muscle on the lateral side of the tibia; upper lateral side of the tibia.

Innervation

Superficial peroneal nerve (L4,L5,S1).

Functional application and strengthening

The peroneus longus muscle passes behind and beneath the lateral malleolus and under the foot from the outside to under the inner surface. Because of its line of pull, it is a strong evertor and assists in plantar flexion.

When the peroneus longus muscle is used effectively with the other ankle flexors, it helps bind the transverse arch as it flexes. Developed without the other plantar flexors, it would produce a weak, everted foot. In running, jumping, hopping, and skipping, the foot should be placed so that it is pointing forward to give proper development of the group. Walking barefoot or in stocking feet on the inside of the foot (everted position) is the best exercise for this muscle.

Eversion exercises may be performed by turning the sole of the foot outward while resistance is applied in the opposite direction to strengthen this muscle.

FIG. 9-11 • Peroneus longus muscle. *O,* Origin; *I,* insertion.

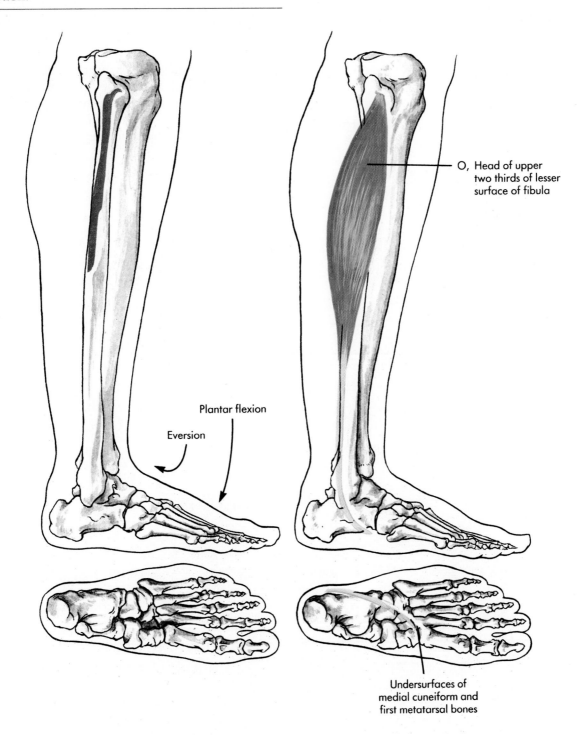

O, Head of upper two thirds of lesser surface of fibula

Plantar flexion

Eversion

Undersurfaces of medial cuneiform and first metatarsal bones

Peroneus brevis muscle FIG. 9-12

(per-o-ne'us bre'vis)

Origin

Lower two thirds of the lateral surface of the fibula.

Insertion

Tuberosity of the fifth metatarsal bone.

Action

Eversion of the foot.
Plantar flexion of the ankle.

Palpation

Tendon of the muscle at the proximal end of the fifth metatarsal.

Innervation

Superficial peroneal nerve (L4,L5,S1).

Functional application and strengthening

The peroneus brevis muscle passes down behind and under the lateral malleolus to pull on the base of the fifth metatarsal. It is a primary evertor of the foot and assists in plantar flexion. In addition, it aids in maintaining the longitudinal arch as it depresses the foot.

The peroneus brevis muscle is exercised with other plantar flexors in the power movements of running, jumping, hopping, and skipping. It may be strengthened in a similar fashion as the peroneus longus by performing eversion exercises such as turning the sole of the foot outward against resistance.

FIG. 9-12 • Peroneus brevis muscle. *O,* Origin; *I,*
insertion.

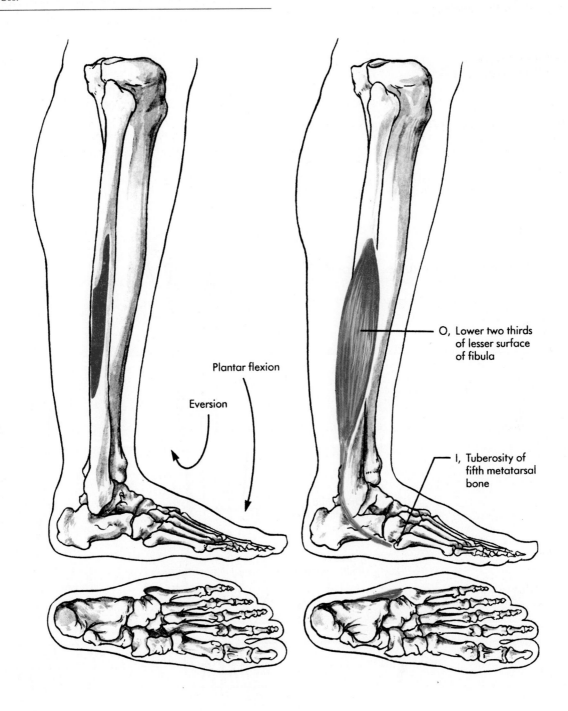

Plantar flexion

Eversion

O, Lower two thirds
of lesser surface
of fibula

I, Tuberosity of
fifth metatarsal
bone

Peroneus tertius muscle FIG. 9-13

(per-o-ne'us ter'shi-us)

Origin

Distal third of the anterior fibula.

Insertion

Base of the fifth metatarsal.

Action

Eversion of the foot.
Dorsal flexion of the ankle.

Palpation

Lateral to the extensor digitorum longus tendon on anterolateral aspect of foot.

Innervation

Deep peroneal nerve (L4, L5, S1).

Functional application and strengthening

The peroneus tertius is a small muscle that assists in dorsal flexion and eversion. It may be strengthened when pulling the foot up toward the shin against a weight or resistance. Everting the foot against resistance such as weighted eversion towel drags can also be used for strength development.

FIG. 9-13 • Peroneus tertius muscle. *O,* Origin; *I,* insertion.

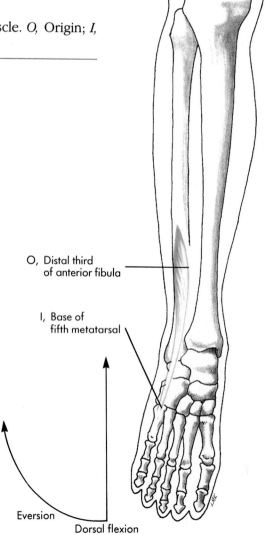
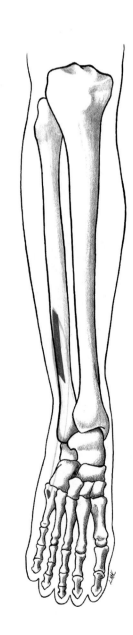

O, Distal third of anterior fibula

I, Base of fifth metatarsal

Eversion

Dorsal flexion

Tibialis anterior muscle FIG. 9-14

(tib-i-a′lis ant-te′ri-or)

Origin

Upper two thirds of the lateral surface of the tibia.

Insertion

Inner surface of the medial cuneiform and the first metatarsal bone.

Action

Dorsal flexion of the ankle.
Inversion of the foot.

Palpation

First muscle to the lateral side of the tibia.

Innervation

Deep peroneal nerve (L4,L5,S1).

FIG. 9-14 • Tibialis anterior muscle. *O,* Origin; *I,* insertion.

Functional application and strengthening

By its insertion, the tibialis anterior muscle is in a fine position to hold up the inner margin of the foot. However, as it contracts, it dorsiflexes the ankle and is used as an antagonist to the plantar flexors of the ankle. The tibialis anterior is forced to contract strongly when a person ice skates or walks on the outside of the foot. It strongly supports the long arch in inversion.

Walking barefoot or in stocking feet on the outside of the foot (inversion) is an excellent exercise for the tibialis anterior muscle.

Turning the sole of the foot to the inside against resistance to perform inversion exercises is one way to strengthen this muscle. Dorsal flexion exercises against resistance may also be used for this purpose.

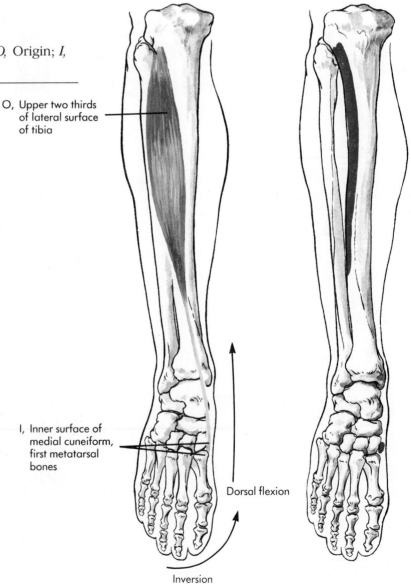

O, Upper two thirds of lateral surface of tibia

I, Inner surface of medial cuneiform, first metatarsal bones

Dorsal flexion

Inversion

Extensor digitorum longus muscle

FIG. 9-15

(eks-ten'sor dij-i-to'rum long'gus)

Origin

Lateral condyle of the tibia, head of the fibula, and upper two thirds of the anterior surface of the fibula.

Insertion

Tops of the middle and distal phalanges of the lesser four toes.

Action

Extension of the four lesser toes.
Dorsal flexion of the ankle.
Eversion of the foot.

Palpation

Second muscle on the lateral side of the tibia; upper lateral side of the tibia.

Innervation

Deep peroneal nerve (L4, L5, S1).

Functional application and strengthening

Strength is necessary in the extensor digitorum longus muscle to maintain balance between the plantar and the dorsal flexors.

Action that involves dorsal flexion of the foot and toes against resistance strengthens both the extensor digitorum longus and the extensor hallucis longus muscles. This may be accomplished by manually applying a downward force on the toes while attempting to extend them up.

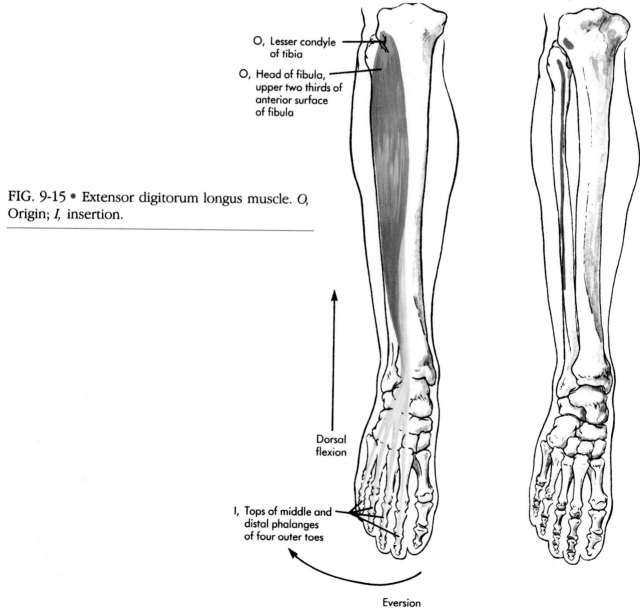

FIG. 9-15 • Extensor digitorum longus muscle. *O,* Origin; *I,* insertion.

O, Lesser condyle of tibia

O, Head of fibula, upper two thirds of anterior surface of fibula

Dorsal flexion

I, Tops of middle and distal phalanges of four outer toes

Eversion

Extensor hallucis longus muscle

FIG. 9-16

(eks-ten'sor hal-u'sis long'gus)

Origin

Middle two thirds of the medial surface of the anterior fibula.

Insertion

Base of the distal phalanx of the great toe.

Action

Dorsiflexion of the ankle.
Extension of the great toe.
Weak inversion of the foot.

Palpation

Near the great toe on the dorsal surface.

Innervation

Deep peroneal nerve (L4, L5, S1).

Functional application and strengthening

The three dorsal flexors of the foot—tibialis anterior, extensor digitorum longus, and extensor hallucis longus—may be exercised by attempting to walk on the heels with the ankle and toes flexed dorsally. Extension of the great toe, as well as ankle dorsiflexion against resistance, will provide strengthening for this muscle.

FIG. 9-16 • Extensor hallucis longus muscle. *O,* Origin; *I,* insertion.

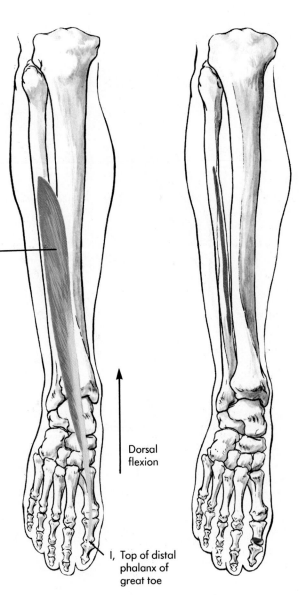

O, Middle two thirds of medial surface of front of fibula

Dorsal flexion

I, Top of distal phalanx of great toe

Muscle identification

In developing a thorough and practical knowledge of the muscular system, it is essential that individual muscles be understood, as well as how groups of muscles work together to produce joint movement (Fig. 9-17).

Intrinsic muscles of the foot

Intrinsic muscles of the foot have their origin and insertion on the bones within the foot. Four layers of these muscles are found on the plantar surface of the foot. The following muscles are found in the four layers.

First layer: Adductor hallucis, flexor digitorum brevis, abductor digiti quinti

Second layer: Quadratus plantae, lumbricales (four)
Third layer: Flexor hallucis brevis, flexor digiti quinti brevis, adductor hallucis
Fourth layer: Interossei (seven)

Muscles are developed and maintain their strength only when they are used. One factor in the great increase in weak foot conditions is the lack of exercise to develop these muscles. Walking is one of the best activities for maintaining and developing these many small muscles that help support the arch of the foot.

Further discussion and consideration of the foot are beyond the scope of this book.

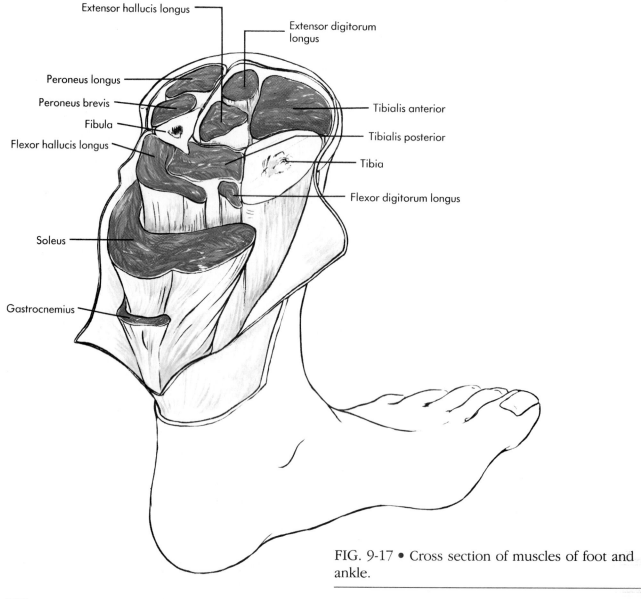

Extensor hallucis longus

Extensor digitorum longus

Peroneus longus

Peroneus brevis

Fibula

Flexor hallucis longus

Tibialis anterior

Tibialis posterior

Tibia

Flexor digitorum longus

Soleus

Gastrocnemius

FIG. 9-17 • Cross section of muscles of foot and ankle.

Worksheet exercises

As an aid to learning, for in-class and out-of-class assignments, or for testing, tearout worksheets are found at the end of the text (p. 226).

Anterior and posterior skeletal worksheet (no. 1)

Draw and label on the worksheet the following muscles of the ankle and foot:
a. Tibialis anterior
b. Extensor digitorum longus
c. Peroneus longus
d. Peroneus brevis
e. Peroneus tertius
f. Soleus
g. Gastrocnemius
h. Extensor hallucis longus
i. Tibialis posterior
j. Flexor digitorum longus
k. Flexor hallucis longus

Laboratory and review exercises

1. Locate the following parts of the ankle and foot on a human skeleton and on a subject:
a. Lateral malleolus
b. Medial malleolus
c. Calcaneus
d. Navicular
e. Three cuneiform bones
f. Metatarsal bones
g. Phalanges

2. How and where do you palpate the following muscles on a human subject?
a. Tibialis anterior
b. Extensor digitorum longus
c. Peroneus longus
d. Peroneus brevis
e. Soleus
f. Gastrocnemius
g. Extensor hallucis longus
h. Flexor digitorum longus
i. Flexor hallucis longus

3. Demonstrate and palpate the following movements:
a. Plantar flexion
b. Dorsal flexion
c. Inversion
d. Eversion
e. Flexion of the toes
f. Extension of the toes

4. Why are "low arches" and "flat feet" not synonymous terms?

5. Discuss the value of proper footwear in various sports and activities.

6. What are orthotics and how do they function?

7. Read and report on some common foot disorders: flat feet, ankle injuries, and hammertoes.

8. Report orally or in writing on magazine articles that rate running and walking shoes.

9. In the chart below, list the muscles primarily responsible for the movements of the ankle, transverse tarsal and subtalar joint, and toes.

Muscle analysis chart • Ankle, transverse tarsal and subtalar joint, and toes

Ankle	
Dorsiflexion	Plantar flexion
Transverse tarsal and subtalar joint	
Eversion	Inversion
Toes	
Flexion	Extension

References

Booher JA, Thibodeau GA: Athletic injury assessment, ed 2, St. Louis, 1989, Mosby.

Dearing M, Ziccardi NJ: Prevention and rehabilitation of ankle injuries, Athletic Journal 66:28, November 1985.

Coughlin LP, et al: Fracture dislocation of the tarsalnavicular: a case report, American Journal of Sports Medicine 15:614, November-December 1987.

Franco AH: Pes cavus and pes planus—analysis and treatment, Physical Therapy 67:688, May 1987.

Grace P: Prevention and rehabilitation of shin splints, Scholastic Coach 57:47, March 1988.

Henderson J: Baring the soles, Runners World 22:14, November 1987.

Robinson M: Feet first, Coach and Athlete 44:30, August-September 1981.

Sammarcho GJ: Foot and ankle injuries in sports (symposium), American Journal of Sports Medicine, November-December 1987.

Sieg KW, Adams SP: Illustrated essentials of musculoskeletal anatomy, ed 2, Gainesville, Fl, 1985, Megabooks.

Stone RJ, Stone JA: Atlas of the skeletal muscles, Dubuque, Iowa, 1990, Brown.

The trunk and spinal column

10

Objectives

- **To identify and differentiate the different types of vertebrae in the spinal column.**

- **To label on a skeletal chart the types of vertebrae and important features.**

- **To draw and label on a skeletal chart some of the muscles of the trunk and the spinal column.**

- **To palpate on a human subject some of the muscles of the trunk and spinal column.**

- **To list and organize the muscles that produce the primary movements of the trunk and spinal column.**

The trunk and thorax present problems in kinesiology that are not found in the study of other parts of the body. First is the complexity of the vertebrae column. It consists of 24 intricate and complex articulating vertebrae. These vertebrae contain the spinal column with its 31 pairs of spinal nerves. Unquestionably it is the most complex part of the human body other than the brain and the central nervous system.

The anterior portion of the trunk contains the abdominal muscles, which are somewhat different from other muscles in that some sections are linked by fascia and tendinous bands and thus do not attach from bone to bone. In addition, the vertebral column contains many small intrinsic muscles, the consideration of which is far beyond the scope of this book.

Bones

Vertebral column FIGS. 10-1 and 10-2

The intricate and complex bony structure of the vertebral column consists of 24 articulating vertebrae and 9 that are fused together. The column is further divided into the cervical (neck) 7 vertebrae, thoracic (chest) 12 vertebrae, and lumbar (lower back) 5 vertebrae. The sacrum (posterior pelvic girdle) and the coccyx (tail bone) consist of 5 and 4 fused vertebrae, respectively. The first two cervical vertebrae are unique in that their shapes allow for extensive rotary movements of the head to the sides, as well as forward and backward. The normal curves of the spine enable it to absorb blows and shocks.

The bones in each region of the spine have slightly different sizes and shapes to allow for various functions. The vertebrae increase in size from the cervical region to the lumbar region primarily because they have to support more weight in the lower back than in the neck. The vertebrae C2 through L5 have similar architecture: they each have a bony block anteriorly, known as the body, a vertebral foramen centrally for the spinal cord to pass through, a transverse process projecting out laterally to each side, and a spinous process projecting posteriorly that is easily palpable.

Thorax

The skeletal foundation of the thorax is formed by 12 pairs of ribs. Seven pairs are true ribs in that they attach directly to the sternum. Five pairs are considered false ribs; three pair attach indirectly to the sternum, and two pairs are floating ribs in that their ends are free. The manubrium, the body of the sternum, and the xiphoid process are the other bones of the thorax. All of the ribs are attached posteriorly to the thoracic vertebrae.

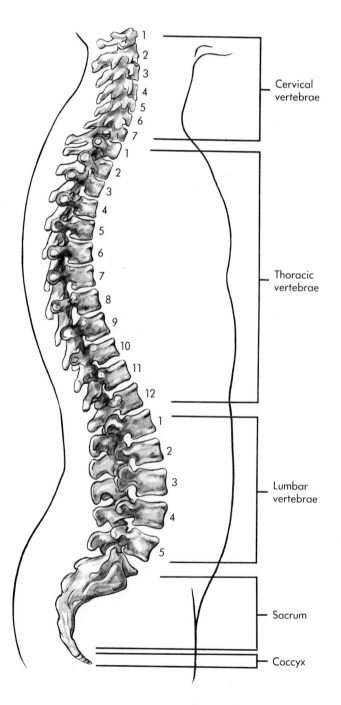

FIG. 10-1 • Vertebral column.

FIG. 10-2 • **A**, Typical cervical vertebra viewed from above; **B**, typical cervical vertebra viewed from the side; **C**, typical thoracic vertebra viewed from above; **D**, typical thoracic vertebra viewed from the side; **E**, third lumbar vertebra viewed from above; **F**, third lumbar vertebra viewed from the side.

From Anthony CP, Kolthoff NJ: Textbook of anatomy and physiology, ed 9, St. Louis, 1975, Mosby.

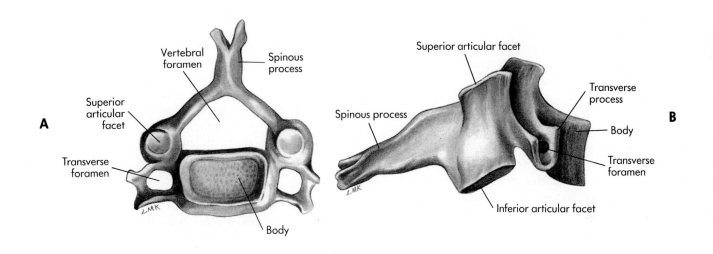

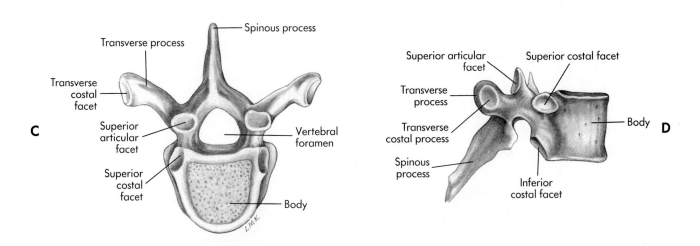

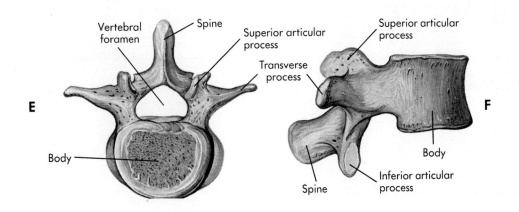

Joints

Except for the atlantoaxial joint formed by the first two cervical vertebrae, there is not a great deal of movement possible between any two vertebrae. However, the cumulative effect of combining the movement from several adjacent vertebrae allows for substantial movements within a given area. Most of the rotation within the cervical region occurs in the atlantoaxial joint, which is classified as a trochoid or pivot-type joint. The remainder of the vertebral articulations are classified as arthodial or gliding-type joints because of their limited gliding movements.

Most of the spinal column movement occurs in the cervical and lumbar regions. There is, of course, some thoracic movement, but it is slight in comparison to that of the neck and low back. In discussing movements of the head, it must be remembered that this movement occurs between the cranium and the first cervical vertebra, as well as within the other cervical vertebrae. With the understanding that these motions usually occur together, for simplification purposes this text refers to all movements of the head and neck as cervical movements. Similarly, in discussing trunk movements, lumbar motion terminology is used to describe the combined motion that occurs in both the thoracic and lumbar regions. A closer investigation of specific motion between any two vertebrae is beyond the scope of this text.

The cervical region can flex 45 degrees and extends 45 degrees. The cervical area laterally flexes 45 degrees and can rotate approximately 60 degrees. The lumbar spine, accounting for most of the trunk movement, flexes approximately 80 degrees and extends 20 to 30 degrees. Lumbar lateral flexion to each side is usually within 35 degrees, and approximately 45 degrees of rotation occur to the left and right.

Movements FIG. 10-3

Spinal movements are often usually preceded by the name given to the region of movement. For example, flexion of the trunk at the lumbar spine is known as lumbar flexion, and extension of the neck is often referred to as cervical extension.

Spinal flexion: anterior movement of the spine; in the cervical region the head moves toward the chest; in the lumbar region the thorax moves toward the pelvis.

Spinal extension: return from flexion or posterior movement of the spine; in the cervical spine the head moves away from the chest; the thorax moves away from the pelvis.

Lateral flexion (left or right): sometimes referred to as side bending; the head moves laterally toward the shoulder; the thorax moves laterally toward the pelvis.

Spinal rotation (left or right): rotary movement of the spine in the horizontal plane; the chin rotates from neutral toward the shoulder; the thorax rotates to one side.

Reduction: return movement from lateral flexion to neutral.

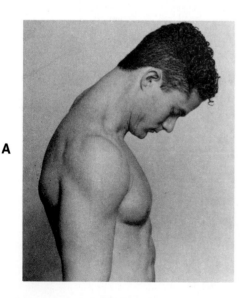
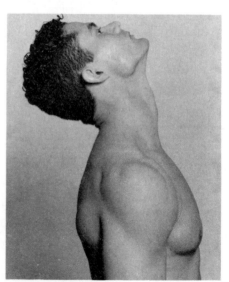

FIG. 10-3 • Movements of the spine. **A,** Cervical flexion; **B,** cervical extension.

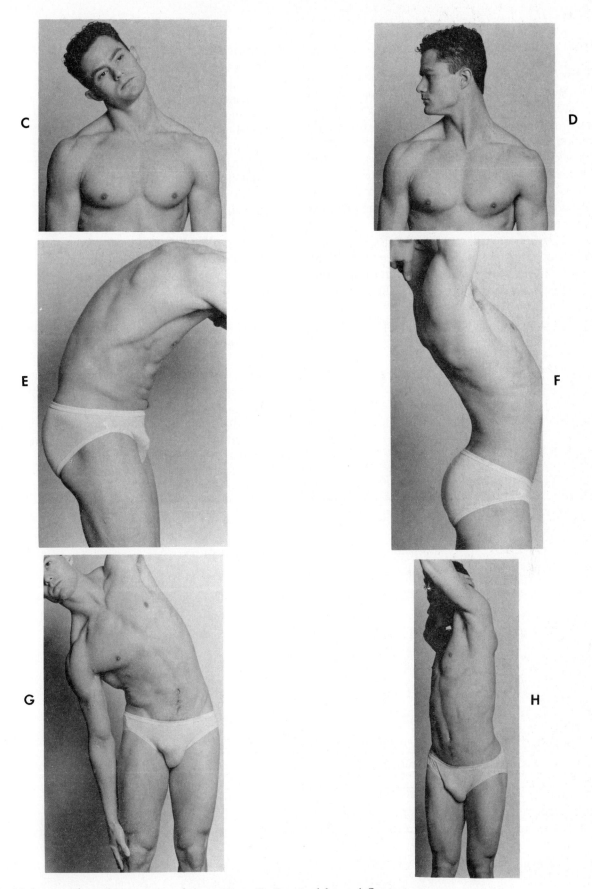

FIG. 10-3 cont'd • Movements of the spine. **C,** Cervical lateral flexion to the right; **D,** cervical rotation to the right; **E,** lumbar flexion; **F,** lumbar extension; **G,** lumbar lateral flexion to the right; **H,** lumbar rotation to the right.

Spinal column muscles

A few large muscles and numerous small muscles are found in this area. The largest muscle is the erector spinae (sacrospinalis), which extends on each side of the spinal column from the pelvic region to the cranium. It is divided into three muscles: the spinalis, the longissimus, and the iliocostalis. From the medial to the lateral side it has attachments in the lumbar, thoracic, and cervical region. Thus the erector spinae group is actually made up of nine muscles.

Numerous small muscles are found in the spinal column region. Many of them have their origin on one vertebra and insertion on the next vertebra. They are important in the functioning of the spine, but knowledge of these muscles is of limited value to most individuals who use this text.

Posterior muscles

Erector spinae (sacrospinalis)
  Spinalis—dorsi, cervicis, capitis
  Longissimus—dorsi, cervicis, capitis
  Iliocostalis—lumborum, dorsi, cervicis
Splenius—capitis and cervicis
Quadratus lumborum
Rotatores—entire spinal column
Multifidus—entire spinal column
Suboccipital
Serratus—superior
Serratus—inferior
Interspinales—entire spinal column
Intertransversales—entire spinal column

Anterior muscles

Some of the anterior muscles are different from other muscles that have been studied. They do not go from bone to bone but attach into an aponeurosis (fascia) around the rectus abdominis area. They are the external oblique abdominal, internal oblique abdominal, and transversus abdominis.

Rectus abdominis
External oblique (obliquus externus abdominis)
Internal oblique (obliquus internus abdominis)
Transversus abdominis

Other anterior and trunk muscles not considered in this text are:

Intercostals—external and internal—from one rib to another
Scaleni
Diaphragm

Rectus abdominis muscle   FIG. 10-4

(rek'tus ab-dom'i-nis)

Origin

Crest of the pubis.

Insertion

Cartilage of the fifth, sixth, and seventh ribs and the xiphoid process.

Action

Both sides: lumbar flexion.
Right side: lateral flexion to the right.
Left side: lateral flexion to the left.

Palpation

Anteromedial surface of the abdomen, between the rib cage and the pubic bone.

Innervation

Intercostal nerves (T7-12).

Functional application and strengthening

The rectus abdominis muscle controls the tilt of the pelvis and the consequent curvature of the lower spine. By holding the pelvis up in front, it flattens the lower back. By pulling the pelvis up in front, it makes the erector spinae muscle more effective as an extensor of the spine and the hip flexors (iliopsoas muscle, particularly) more effective in raising the legs.

There are several exercises for the abdominal muscles such as leg raises, straight-leg sit-ups, bent-knee sit-ups, crunches, and isometric contractions. Bent-knee sit-ups with the arms folded across the chest are considered by many to be a safe and efficient exercise. Crunches are also considered to be very effective for isolating the work to the abdominals. Both of these exercises largely eliminate the action of the iliopsoas muscle and other hip flexors by shortening them, thus reducing their ability to generate force. Twisting to the left and right brings the oblique muscles into more active contraction.

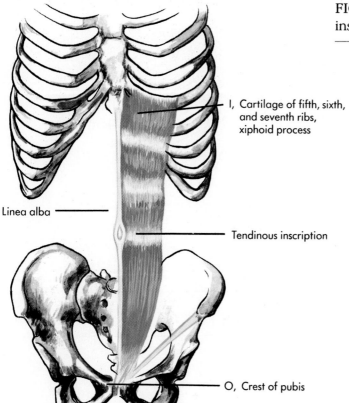

FIG. 10-4 ● Rectus abdominis muscle. *O,* Origin; *I,* insertion.

I, Cartilage of fifth, sixth, and seventh ribs, xiphoid process

Linea alba

Tendinous inscription

O, Crest of pubis

External oblique abdominal muscle

FIG. 10-5

(ik-stur'nel o-blek' ab-dom'i-nel)

Origin

Borders of the lower eight ribs at the side of the chest dove-tailing with the serratus anterior muscle.*

Insertion

Anterior half of the crest of the ilium, the inguinal ligament, the crest of pubis, and the fascia of the rectus abdominis muscle at the lower front.

Action

Both sides: lumbar flexion.

Right side: lumbar lateral flexion to the right and rotation to the left.

Left side: lumbar lateral flexion to the left and rotation to the right.

---

*Sometimes the origin and insertion are reversed in anatomy books. This is the result of different interpretations of which bony structure is the more movable. The insertion is considered the most movable part of a muscle.

Palpation

Lateral side of the abdomen, either left or right.

Innervation

Intercostal nerves (T8-12), iliohypogastric nerve (T12, L1), and ilioinguinal nerve (L1).

Functional application and strengthening

Working on each side of the abdomen, the external oblique abdominal muscles aid in rotating the trunk when working independently of each other. Working together, they aid the rectus abdominis muscle in its described action. The left external oblique abdominal muscle comes strongly into contraction during sit-ups when the trunk rotates to the right, as in touching the left elbow to the right knee. Rotating to the left brings the right external oblique into action.

FIG. 10-5 • External oblique abdominal muscle. *O,* Origin; *I,* insertion.

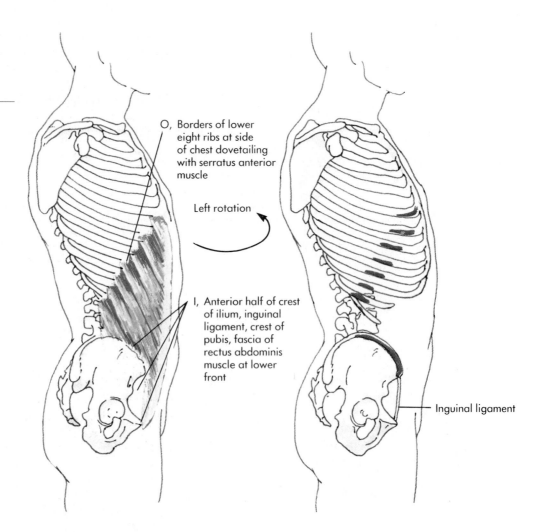

O, Borders of lower eight ribs at side of chest dovetailing with serratus anterior muscle

Left rotation

I, Anterior half of crest of ilium, inguinal ligament, crest of pubis, fascia of rectus abdominis muscle at lower front

Inguinal ligament

Internal oblique abdominal muscle

FIG. 10-6

(ik-stur′nel o-blek″ ab-dom′i-nel)

Origin

Upper half of the inguinal ligament, anterior two thirds of the crest of the ilium, and the lumbar fascia.

Insertion

Costal cartilages of the eighth, ninth, and tenth ribs and the linea alba.

Action

Both sides: lumbar flexion.
Right side: lumbar lateral flexion and rotation to the right.
Left side: lumbar lateral flexion and rotation to the left.

Palpation

Palpated on the lateral side of the abdomen when the external oblique is relaxed.

Innervation

Intercostal nerves (T8-12), iliohypogastric nerve (T12, L1), and ilioinguinal nerve (L1).

Functional application and strengthening

The internal oblique abdominal muscles run diagonally in the direction opposite to that of the external oblique. The left internal oblique rotates to the left, and the right internal oblique rotates to the right.

In touching the left elbow to the right knee in sit-ups, the left external oblique and the right internal oblique abdominal muscles rotate at the same time, assisting the rectus abdominis muscle in flexing the trunk to make the completion of the movement possible. In rotary movements the internal oblique and the external oblique on opposite sides from each other always work together.

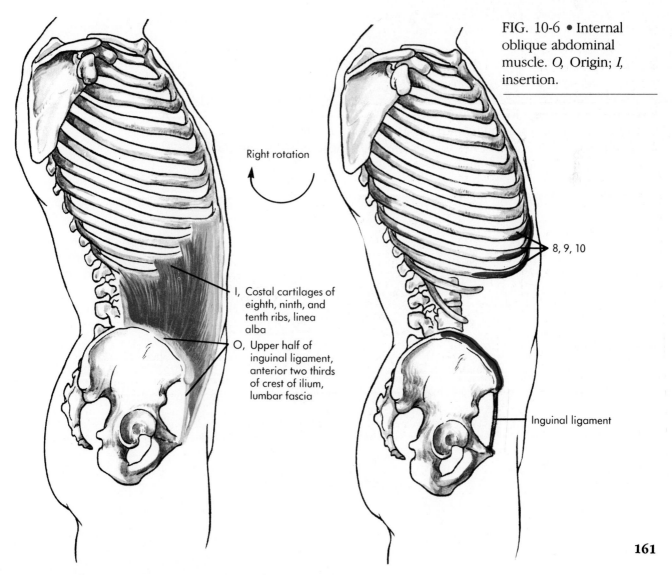

FIG. 10-6 • Internal oblique abdominal muscle. *O,* Origin; *I,* insertion.

Right rotation

I, Costal cartilages of eighth, ninth, and tenth ribs, linea alba

O, Upper half of inguinal ligament, anterior two thirds of crest of ilium, lumbar fascia

8, 9, 10

Inguinal ligament

161

Transverse abdominis muscle

FIGS. 10-7 and 10-8

(trans-vurs′ ab-dom′i-nis)

Origin

Outer third of the inguinal ligament.
Inner rim of the iliac crest.
Inner surface of the cartilage of the lower six ribs.
Lumbar fascia.

Insertion

Crest of the pubis and the iliopectineal line.
Abdominal aponeurosis to linea alba.

Action

Forced expiration by pulling the abdominal wall inward.

Palpation

Cannot be palpated.

Innervation

Intercostal nerves (T7-12), iliohypogastric nerve (T12, L1), and ilioinguinal nerve (L1).

Functional application and strengthening

The transversus abdominis is the chief muscle of forced expiration and is effective, together with the rectus abdominis, the external oblique abdominal, and the internal oblique abdominal muscles, in helping to hold the abdomen flat.

The transversus abdominis muscle is exercised effectively by attempting to draw the abdominal contents back toward the spine. This may be done isometrically in the supine position or while standing.

FIG. 10-7 • Abdominal wall. Unique arrangement of four abdominal muscles with their fascial attachment in and around rectus abdominis muscle is shown. With no bones for attachments, these muscles can be adequately maintained through exercise.

Modified from Anthony CP, Kolthoff NH: Textbook of anatomy and physiology, ed 9, St. Louis, 1975, Mosby.

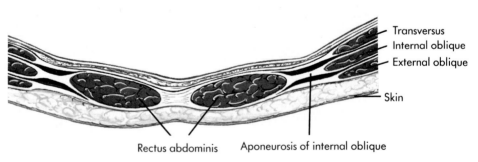

Transversus
Internal oblique
External oblique
Skin
Rectus abdominis   Aponeurosis of internal oblique

FIG. 10-8 • Transversus abdominis muscle. *O*, Origin; *I*, insertion.

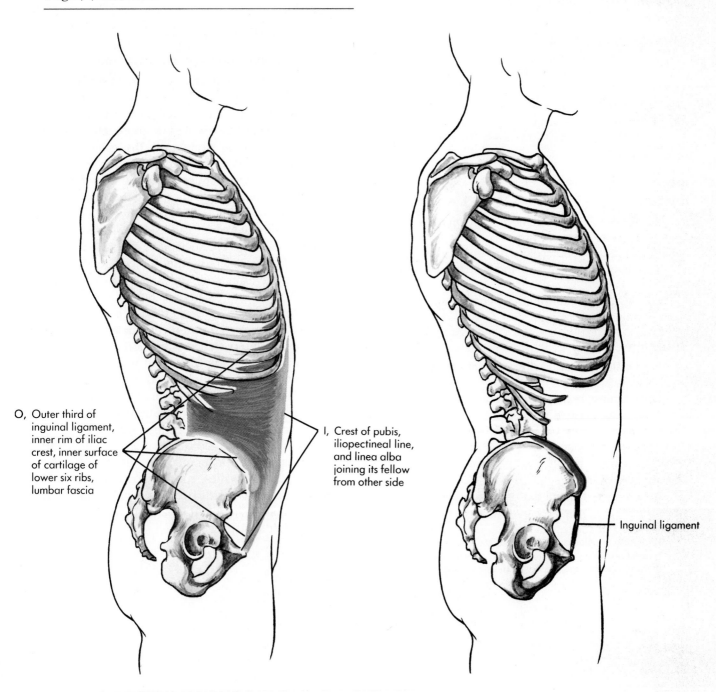

O, Outer third of inguinal ligament, inner rim of iliac crest, inner surface of cartilage of lower six ribs, lumbar fascia

I, Crest of pubis, iliopectineal line, and linea alba joining its fellow from other side

Inguinal ligament

Erector spinae muscle*
(sacrospinalis) FIG. 10-9
(e-rek'tor spi'ne) (sa'kro-spi-na'lis)

Iliocostalis
(il'i-o-kos-ta'lis): lateral layer

Longissimus
(lon-jis'i-mus): middle layer

Spinalis
(spi-na'lis): medial layer

Origin

Iliocostalis: Thoracolumbar aponeurosis from sacrum, posterior ribs.

Longissimus: Thoracolumbar aponeurosis from sacrum, lumbar and thoracic transverse processes.

Spinalis: ligamentum nuchae, cervical and thoracic spinous processes.

Insertion

Iliocostalis: posterior ribs, cervical transverse processes.

Longissimus: cervical and thoracic transverse processes, mastoid process.

Spinalis: cervical and thoracic spinous processes, occipital bone.

Action

Extension and lateral flexion of the spine.

---

*This muscle includes the iliocostalis, the longissimus dorsi, the spinalis dorsi, and divisions of these muscles in the lumbar, thoracic, and cervical sections of the spinal column.

Palpation

Lower lumbar region on either side of the spine.

Innervation

Posterior branches of spinal nerves.

Functional application and strengthening

The erector spinae muscle functions best when the pelvis is held up in front, thus pulling it down slightly in back. This lowers the origin of the erector spinae and makes it more effective in keeping the spine straight. As the spine is held straight, the ribs are raised, thus fixing the chest high and consequently making the abdominal muscles more effective in holding the pelvis up in front and flattening the abdominal wall.

An exercise known as "dead lift," employing a barbell, uses the erector spinae in extending the spine. In this exercise the subject bends over, keeping the arms and legs straight, picks up the barbell, and returns to a standing position. In performing this type of exercise, it is very important to always use correct technique to avoid back injuries. Voluntary static contraction of the erector spinae in the standing position would provide a mild exercise and improve body posture.

The erector spinae and its various divisions may be strengthened through numerous forms of back extension exercises. These are usually done in a prone or face-down position in which the spine is already in some state of flexion. The subject then uses these muscles to move part or all of the spine toward extension against gravity. A weight may be held in the hands behind the head to increase resistance.

FIG. 10-9 • Erector spinae (sacrospinalis) muscle.
A, Iliocostalis; **B**, longissimus; **C**, spinalis.

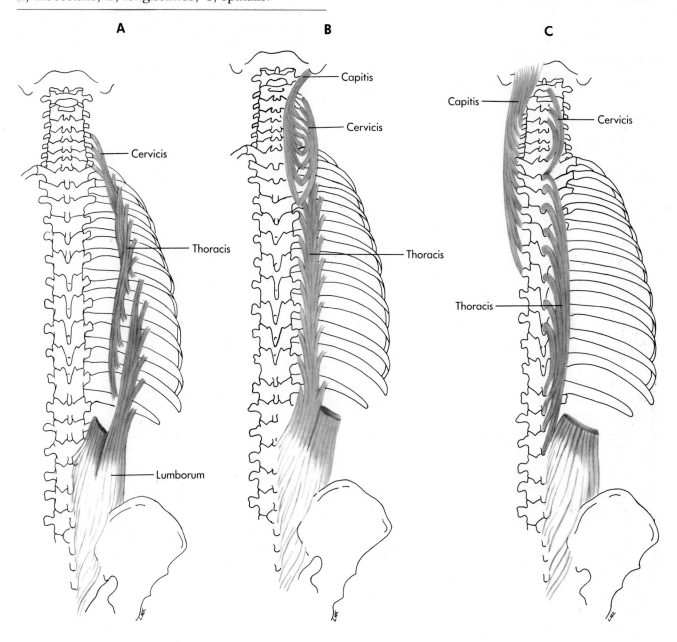

A

Cervicis

Thoracis

Lumborum

B

Capitis

Cervicis

Thoracis

C

Capitis

Cervicis

Thoracis

Quadratus lumborum muscle FIG. 10-10

(kwad-ra′tus lum-bo′rum)

Origin

Posterior inner lip of the iliac crest.

Insertion

Transverse processes of the upper four lumbar vertebrae and lower border of the twelfth rib.

Action

Lateral flexion to the side on which it is located. Stabilizes the pelvis and lumbar spine.

Palpation

For all practical purposes, it is impossible to palpate except on an extremely thin individual.

Innervation

Branches of T12, L1 nerves.

Functional application and strengthening

The quadratus lumborum is important in lumbar lateral flexion and in elevating the pelvis on the same side in the standing position. Trunk rotation and lateral flexion movements against resistance are good exercises for development of this muscle. The position of the body relative to gravity may be changed to increase resistance on this and other trunk and abdominal muscles.

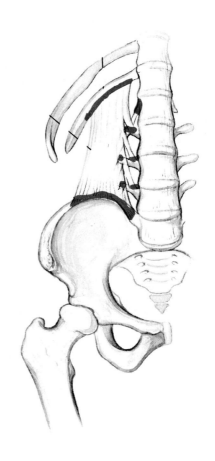

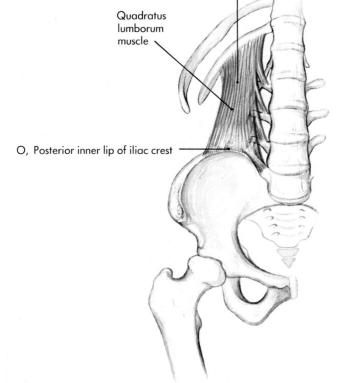

I, Transverse processes of upper four lumbar vertebrae and lower border of twelfth rib

Quadratus lumborum muscle

O, Posterior inner lip of iliac crest

FIG. 10-10 • Quadratus lumborum muscle. *O,* Origin; *I,* insertion.

Modified from Anthony CP, Kolthoff NJ: Textbook of anatomy and physiology, ed 9, St. Louis, 1975, Mosby.

Splenius muscles (cervicis, capitis)

FIG. 10-11

(sple′ni-us) (ser′vi-sis) (kap′i-tis)

Origin

Splenius cervicis: spinous processes of the third through the sixth thoracic vertebrae.

Splenius capitis: lower half of the ligamentum nuchae and the spinous processes of the seventh cervical and the upper three or four thoracic vertebrae.

Insertion

Splenius cervicis: transverse processes of the first three cervical vertebrae.

Splenius capitis: mastoid process and occipital bone.

Action

Both sides: extension of the head and neck.
Right side: rotation and lateral flexion to the right.
Left side: rotation and lateral flexion to the left.

Palpation

Cannot be palpated.

Innervation

Posterior lateral branches of cervical nerves four through eight (C4-8).

Functional application and strengthening

Any movement of the head and neck into extension, particularly extension and rotation, would bring the splenius muscle strongly into play, together with the erector spinae and the upper trapezius muscles. Tone in the splenius muscle tends to hold the head and neck in proper posture position.

A good exercise for the splenius muscle is to lace the fingers behind the head with the muscle in flexion and then to slowly contract the posterior head and neck muscles to move the head and neck into full extension. This exercise may also be performed by using a towel or a partner for resistance.

FIG. 10-11 • Splenius muscles (cervicis on the left, capitis on the right). *O,* Origin; *I,* insertion.

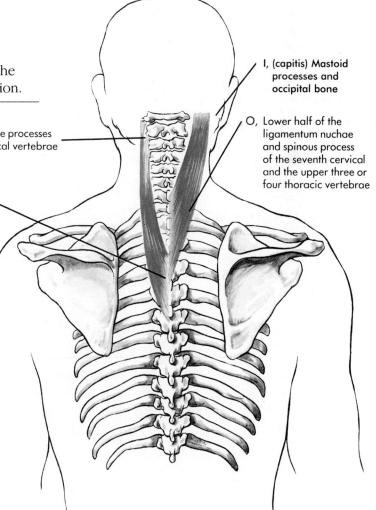

I, (cervicis) Transverse processes of first three cervical vertebrae

O, Spinous processes of the third through sixth thoracic vertebrae

I, (capitis) Mastoid processes and occipital bone

O, Lower half of the ligamentum nuchae and spinous process of the seventh cervical and the upper three or four thoracic vertebrae

Sternocleidomastoid muscle FIG. 10-12

(ster′no-kli-do-mas-toyd)

Origin

Manubrium of the sternum.
Medial clavicle.

Insertion

Mastoid process.

Action

Both sides: cervical flexion.
Right side: rotation to the left and lateral flexion to
the right.
Left side: rotation to the right and lateral flexion to
the left.

Palpation

Anterolateral neck, diagonally between the origin and
insertion.

FIG. 10-12 • Sternocleidomastoid muscle, anterior
view. *O*, Origin; *I*, insertion.

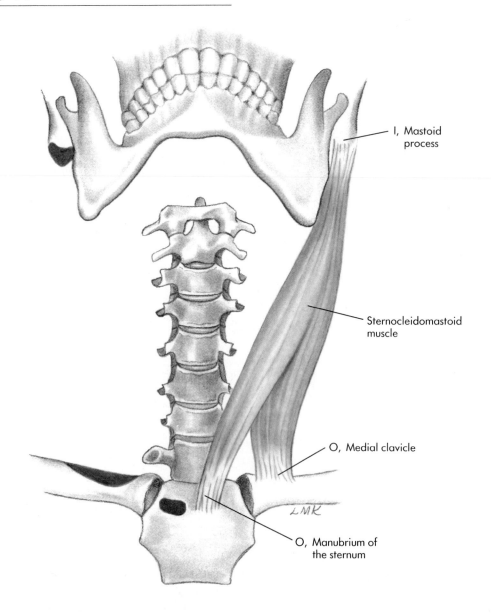

I, Mastoid
process

Sternocleidomastoid
muscle

O, Medial clavicle

O, Manubrium of
the sternum

Innervation

Spinal accessory nerve (Cr11, C2-3).

Functional application and strengthening

The sternocleidomastoid is primarily responsible for flexion and rotation of the head and neck. One side of this muscle may be easily visualized and palpated when rotating the head to the opposite side.

The sternocleidomastoid is easily worked for strength development by placing the hands on the forehead to apply force posteriorly while using these muscles to pull the head forward into flexion. The hand may also be used on one side of the jaw to apply rotary force in the opposite direction while the sternocleidomastoid is contracting concentrically to rotate the head in the direction of the hand.

FIG. 10-12 cont'd • Sternocleidomastoid muscle, lateral view.

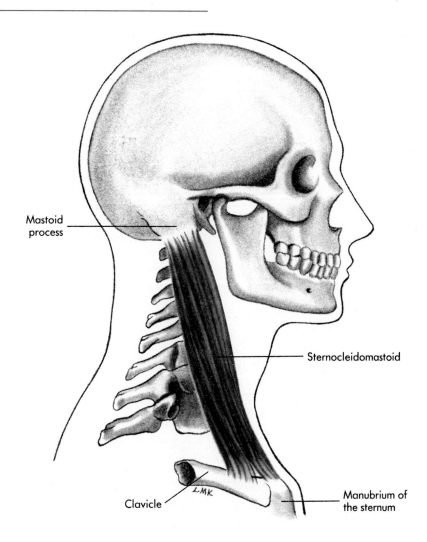

Mastoid process

Sternocleidomastoid

Clavicle

Manubrium of the sternum

Worksheet exercises

As an aid to learning, for in-class and out-of-class assignments, or for testing, tearout worksheets are found at the end of the text (pp. 227 and 228).

Anterior skeletal worksheet (no. 1)

Draw and label the following muscles on the skeletal chart:
a. Rectus abdominus
b. External oblique abdominal
c. Internal oblique abdominal

Posterior skeletal worksheet (no. 2)

Draw and label the following muscles on the skeletal chart:
a. Erector spinae
b. Quadrus lumborum
c. Splenius—cervicis and capitis

Laboratory and review exercises

1. Locate the following parts of the spine on a human skeleton and human subject:
   a. Cervical vertebrae
   b. Thoracic vertebrae
   c. Lumbar vertebra
   d. Spinous processes
   e. Transverse processes
   f. Sacrum
   g. Manubrium
   h. Xiphoid process
   i. Sternum
   j. Rib cage (various ribs)
2. How and where do you palpate the following muscles on a human subject?
   a. Rectus abdominis
   b. External oblique abdominal
   c. Internal oblique abdominal
   d. Erector spinae
   e. Sternocleidomastoid
3. Contrast crunches with bent-knee sit-ups and with straight-leg sit-ups. Does having a partner to hold the feet make a difference in the ability to do the bent-knee and straight-leg sit-ups? If so, why?
4. Which exercise is better for the development of the abdominal muscles—leg-lifts or sit-ups? Defend your answer.
5. Why is good abdominal muscular development so important? Why is this area so frequently neglected?
6. Why are weak abdominal muscles frequently blamed for lower back pains?
7. Prepare an oral or written report on abdominal or back injuries found in the literature.
8. Fill in the movements and muscle actions of the cervical and lumbar spine on the chart on the next page. List the muscles primarily responsible for each movement.

Muscle analysis chart • Lumbar and cervical spine

Cervical spine	
Flexion	Extension
Lateral flexion right	Rotation right
Lateral flexion left	Rotation left

Lumbar spine	
Flexion	Extension
Lateral flexion right	Rotation right
Lateral flexion left	Rotation left

References

Clarkson HM, Gilewich GB: Musculoskeletal assessment: joint range of motion and manual muscle strength, Baltimore, 1989, Williams & Wilkins.

Daniels L, Worthingham C: Muscle testing: techniques of manual examination, ed 5, Philadelphia, 1986, Saunders.

Day AL: Observation on the treatment of lumbar disc disease in college football players, American Journal of Sports Medicine, 15:7275, January-February 1987.

Holden DL, Jackson DW: Stress fractures of ribs in female rowers, American Journal of Sports Medicine, 13:277, July-August 1987.

Martens MA, et al: Adductor tendonitus and muscular abdominis tendopathy, American Journal of Sports Medicine, 15:353, July-August 1987.

Marymont JV: Exercise-related stress reaction of the sacrilian joint, an unusual cause of low back pain in athletes, American Journal of Sports Medicine, 14:320, July-August 1986.

Rasch PJ: Kinesiology and applied anatomy, ed 7, 1989, Philadelphia, Lea & Febiger.

Sieg KW, Adams SP: Illustrated essentials of musculoskeletal anatomy, ed 2, Gainesville, Fl, 1985, Megabooks.

Stone RJ, Stone JA: Atlas of the skeletal muscles, Dubuque, IA, 1990, Brown.

Muscular analysis of selected exercises and activities

11

. . . .

Objectives

- **To understand various conditioning principles and how to apply them to strengthening major muscle groups.**

- **To know and understand the different types of muscle contractions.**

- **To learn to analyze an exercise for the types of contractions occurring in specific muscles to create major joint movements.**

- **To learn to analyze and prescribe exercises to strengthen all major muscle groups.**

Chapter 6 presented an introduction to the analysis of exercise and activities. That chapter included only the analysis of the muscles previously studied in the upper extremity region.

Since that chapter, all the other joints and large muscle groups of the human body have been considered. The exercises and activities found in this chapter consider muscles in other parts of the body and analyze further the upper extremity muscles.

Strength, endurance, and flexibility of the muscles of the lower extremity, trunk, and abdominal sections are also very important in skillful physical performance and body maintenance.

The type of contraction is determined by whether the muscle is lengthening or shortening during the movement. However, muscles may shorten or lengthen in the absence of a contraction through passive movement caused by other contracting muscles, momentum, gravity, or external forces such as manual assistance machines.

Concentric contraction is a shortening contraction of the muscles against gravity or resistance, whereas eccentric contraction is a condition in which the muscle lengthens under tension to control the joints moving with gravity or resistance.

Contraction against gravity is also quite evident in the lower extremities.

The quadriceps muscle group contracts eccentrically when the body slowly lowers in a weight-bearing movement through lower extremity action. The quadriceps functions as a decelerator to knee joint flexion in weight-bearing movments by contracting eccentrically to prevent too rapid a downward movement. One can easily demonstrate this fact by palpating this muscle group when slowly moving from a standing position to a half squat. Almost as much work is done in this type of contraction as in concentric contractions.

In this example involving the quadriceps, the slow descent is eccentric, and the ascent from the squatted position is concentric. If the descent were at the same speed as gravity, essentially under no muscular control, the muscle lengthening would be passive. That is, the movement and change in length of the muscle would be caused by gravity and not by active muscular contractions.

In recent years more and more muscle educators on all levels have been emphasizing the development of local muscle groups through resistance training and circuit-training activities.

Athletes and nonathletes, both male and female, need to have overall muscular development.

Sport participation does not ensure sufficient development of local muscle groups. Also, more and more emphasis has been placed on mechanical kinesiology in physical education and athletic skill teaching. This is desirable and can help bring about more skillful performance, but one must remember that mechanical principles will be of little or no value to performers without adequate strength and endurance of their muscular system, which is developed through planned exercises and activities. In the fitness and health revolution of recent years, a much greater emphasis has been placed on exercises and activites that improve the physical fitness, strength, endurance, and flexibility of participants. This chapter will continue the practice of analyzing the muscles through simple exercises that began in Chapter 6. When these techniques are mastered, the individual is ready to analyze and prescribe exercises and activities for muscular strength and endurance needed in sport activities and for healthful living.

Conditioning considerations

Overload principle

A basic physiological principle of exercise is the overload principle. It states that a muscle or muscle group increases in strength in direct proportion to the overload placed on it. To improve the strength and functioning of major muscles, muscle educators need to apply this principle to every large muscle group in the body, progressively throughout each year, at all age levels. Increasing the speed of doing the exercise, the number of repetitions, the weight, and more bouts of exercise are all ways to apply this principle.

Many coaches are having their athletes perform various weight-training activities (overload principle) during the season to maintain and improve the strength of muscle groups.

SAID principle

The SAID (**S**pecific **A**daptations to **I**mposed **De**mands) principle should be considered in all aspects of physiological conditioning and training. This principle, which states that the body will gradually, over time, adapt very specifically to the various stresses and overloads to which it is subjected, is applicable in every form of muscle training.

It should be recognized that this adaptation may be positive or negative, depending on whether or not the correct techniques are used and stressed in the design and administration of the conditioning program. Inappropriate or excessive demands placed on the body in too short of a time span can result in injury. If the demands are too minimal or administered too infrequently over too long a time period, less than desired improvement will occur. Conditioning programs and the exercises included in them should be analyzed to determine if they are usng the specific muscles for which they were intended in the correct manner.

Specificity

The specific needs of the individual must be specifically addressed when designing an exercise program. Quite often, it will be necessary to analyze an individual's exercise and skill technique to specifically design an exercise program to meet his or her needs. Potential exercises to be used in the conditioning program must be analyzed to determine their appropriateness for the individual's specific needs. Regular observation and follow-up exercise analysis is necessary to ensure proper adherence to correct technique.

Analysis of movement

When analyzing various exercises and sport skills, it is essential to break down all of the movements into phases. The number of phases, usually three to five, will vary, depending on the skill. Practically all sport skills will have at least a preparatory phase, a movement phase, and a follow-through phase, whereas many will begin with a stance phase and end with a recovery phase. The names of the phases will vary from skill to skill to fit in with the terminology used in various sports.

The *stance* phase allows the athlete to assume a comfortable and balanced body position from which to initiate the sport skill. The emphasis is on setting the various joint angles in the correct positions in respect to one another and the sport surface.

The *preparatory* phase, often referred to as the cocking or wind-up phase, is used to lengthen the appropriate muscles so that they will be in position to generate more force and momentum as they concentrically contract in the next phase.

The *movement* phase, sometimes known as the acceleration, action, motion, or contact phase, is the action part of the skill. It is the phase in which the summation of force is generated directly to the ball, sport object, opponent, etc. and is usually characterized by near maximal concentric activity in the involved muscles.

The *follow-through* phase begins immediately after the climax of the movement phase in order to bring about negative acceleration of the involved limb or body segment. In this phase, often referred to as the deceleration phase, the velocity of the body segment progressively decreases usually over a wide range of motion.

This velocity decrease is usually attributable to high eccentric activity in the involved muscles.

The *recovery* phase is used after follow-through to regain balance and positioning to be ready for the next sport demand.

Skill analysis can be seen with the example of a tennis serve. The stance phase begins when the player assumes a position with the ball hand facing the net immediately before tossing the ball into the air. As the ball is thrown into the air, the racket arm and shoulder are cocked back into the preparatory phase, followed very quickly by the movement phase to bring the arm forward so the racket can make contact with the ball. The racket arm continues moving in the same direction established by the movement phase until the velocity decreases to the point that the arm can safely change movement direction. At this point, the recovery phase begins, enabling the player to reposition to meet the opponent's return of the serve. In this example reference has been made briefly only to the racket arm, but in actual practice the movements of each joint in the body should be analyzed into the various phases.

Muscular development

For years it was thought that a person developed adequate muscular strength through participation in sport activities. Now the philosophy is that one develops muscular strength to be able to adequately participate in sport activities.

Adequate muscular strength of the entire body from head to toe should be developed. Individuals responsible for this development need to prescribe exercises that will meet this objective.

In schools this development should start at an early age and continue throughout the school years. Results of fitness tests have found that there is need for considerable improvement in this area. The chin-up (pull-up) test had to be modified because more that 50% of children could not do one chin-up. Sit-ups, the standing long jump, the mile run, and other tests all indicated fitness deficiencies in the children of the United States. Adequate muscular strength and endurance are important in the adult years. Many back pains and other physical ailments could be avoided through proper maintenance of the musculoskeletal system.

The exercises in this chapter will help individuals learn how to analyze and prescribe exercises for overall muscular development for young and old.

Sit-up—bent knee

Description

The subject lies on the back, fingers interlaced behind the neck, with the knees flexed approximately 90 degrees and the feet about hip-width apart.

The subject curls up to a sitting position, twists the trunk to the left, touches the right elbow to the left knee, and then returns to the starting position.

Analysis

This exercise is divided into four movements for analysis: (1) curling movement to sitting-up position, (2) twisting movement to left, (3) return movement to sitting-up position, and (4) return movement to starting position.

Curling movement to sitting-up position
Trunk
- Flexion
  - Rectus abdominis
  - External oblique abdominal
  - Internal oblique abdominal

Hip
- Flexion
  - Illiopsoas
  - Rectus femoris
  - Pectineus

Twisting movement to left
Trunk
- Left lateral rotation and flexion
  - Left rectus abdominis
  - Right external oblique abdominal
  - Left internal oblique abdominal
  - Left erector spinae

Right shoulder girdle
- Abduction
  - Serratus anterior
  - Pectoralis minor

Left shoulder girdle
- Adduction
  - Trapezius
  - Rhomboid

Right shoulder joint
- Horizontal adduction
  - Pectoralis major
  - Anterior deltoid
  - Coracobrachialis

Left shoulder joint
- Horizontal abduction
  - Posterior deltoid
  - Infraspinatus
  - Teres minor
  - Latissimus dorsi

Return movement to sitting-up position
Trunk
- Right lateral rotation and flexion
  - Right rectus abdominis
  - Left external oblique abdominal
  - Right internal oblique abdominal
  - Right erector spinae

Right shoulder girdle
- Adduction
  - Rhomboid
  - Trapezius

Left shoulder girdle
- Abduction
  - Serratus anterior
  - Pectoralis minor

Right shoulder joint
- Horizontal abduction
  - Posterior deltoid
  - Infraspinatus
  - Teres minor
  - Latissimus dorsi

Left shoulder joint
- Horizontal adduction
  - Pectoralis major
  - Anterior deltoid
  - Coracobrachialis

Return movement to starting position
Trunk
- Extension—trunk flexors (eccentric contraction)
  - Rectus abdominis
  - External oblique abdominal
  - Internal oblique abdominal

Hip
- Extension—hip flexors (eccentric contraction)
  - Illiopsoas
  - Rectus femoris
  - Pectineus

Prone arch FIG. 11-1

Description

The subject lies in a prone position, face down, with the arms in an adducted and relaxed position lying beside the body. The head, upper trunk, and legs are raised from the floor. The legs are kept straight. Then the subject returns to the starting position.

Analysis

This exercise is separated into two movements for analysis: (1) movement to raise head, trunk, and legs; and (2) return movement to starting position.

Movement to raise head, trunk, and legs
  Trunk and head
    Extension
    Erector spinae
    Splenius
    Quadratus lumborum

Hip
  Extension
    Gluteus maximus
    Semitendinosus
    Semimembranosus
    Biceps femoris
Return movement to starting position
  Trunk and head
    Flexion (return to neutral flat position)
      Trunk and head extensors (eccentric contraction)
        Erector spinae
        Splenius
        Quadratus lumborum
Hip
    Flexion (return to neutral flat position)
      Hip extensors (eccentric contraction)
        Gluteus maximus
        Semitendinosus
        Semimembranosus
        Biceps femoris

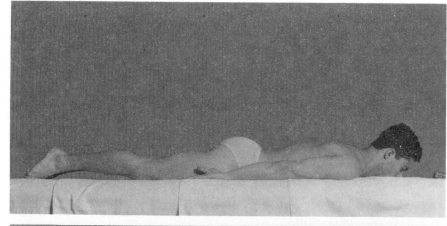

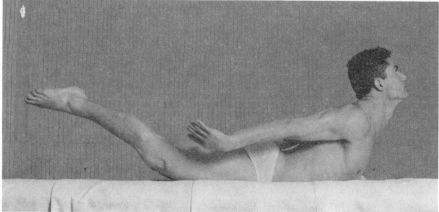

FIG. 11-1 • Prone arch. **A**, Beginning relaxed position; **B**, fully arched position.

FREE WEIGHT-TRAINING EXERCISES*

Exercise through the use of weights has become increasingly important as a means of developing and maintaining muscular strength in young people and adults. When this type of exercise is undertaken, a thorough knowledge of the muscles being used is essential so that one group of muscles is not overdeveloped and another underdeveloped.

Most schools have free weights, barbells, and dumbells available for use by students. Some physical education teachers and coaches recommend that junior and senior high school students have their own barbell set for use at home.

An analysis of several selected weight-training exercises will introduce the muscular analysis of these activities. In these exercises the only equipment needed is a barbell with weights.

---

*These are only sample weight-training exercises. Students are encouraged to continue the study of muscular analysis of the many other weight-training exercises and activities.

Arm curl

Description

With the subject in a standing position, the barbell is held in the hands with the palms to the front. The barbell is curled upward and forward until the elbows are completely flexed. Then it is returned to the starting position.

Analysis

This exercise is divided into two movements for analysis: (1) upward curl movement, and (2) return movement to starting position. NOTE: An assumption is made that no movement occurs in the shoulder joint and shoulder girdle.

Upward curl movement

  Wrist and hand (The finger flexors remain contracted throughout the entire exercise to hold the bar)

  Flexion

    Flexor carpi radialis

    Flexor carpi ulnaris

    Palmaris longus

    Flexor digitorum profundus

    Flexor digitorum superficialis

    Flexor pollicis longus

  Elbow joint

  Flexion

  Biceps brachii

  Brachialis

  Brachioradialis

Return movement to starting position

  Wrist and hand (wrist only, not fingers)

  Extension (eccentric contraction)

    Flexor carpi radialis

    Flexor carpi ulnaris

    Palmaris longus

    Flexor digitorum profundus

    Flexor digitorum superficialis

    Flexor pollicis longus

  Elbow joint

  Extension (eccentric contraction)

    Biceps brachii

    Brachialis

    Brachioradialis

Barbell press FIG. 11-2

Description

This exercise is sometimes referred to as the overhead or military press. The barbell is held in a position high in front of the chest with palms facing forward, feet comfortably spread, and back and legs straight. From this position it is pushed upward until the arms are fully flexed overhead, and then it is returned to the starting position.

Analysis

This exercise is separated into two movements for analysis: (1) upward movement, and (2) return movement to starting position.

Upward curl movement
Wrist and hand
No movement
Wrist and hand flexors (isometric contraction)
Elbow joint
Extension
Triceps brachii
Anconeus

Shoulder joint
Flexion
Pectoralis major (clavicular head—upper fibers)
Anterior deltoid
Coracobrachialis
Biceps brachii
Shoulder girdle
Upward rotation and elevation
Trapezius
Levator scapulae
Serratus anterior
Return movement to starting position
Wrist and hand
No movement
Elbow joint
Flexion
Elbow joint extensors (eccentric contraction)
Shoulder joint
Extension
Shoulder joint flexors (eccentric contraction)
Shoulder girdle
Downward rotation and depression
Shoulder girdle upward rotators and elevators (eccentric contraction)

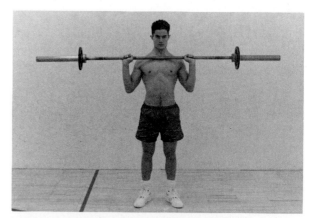

A

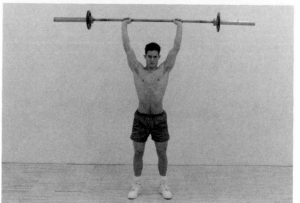

B

FIG. 11-2 • Barbell press. **A**, Starting position; **B**, full overhead position.

Squat FIG. 11-3

Description

The subject places a barbell on the shoulders behind the neck and grasps it with the palms-forward position of the hands. He squats down until the thighs are parallel to the floor, keeping the back straight, and then returns to the starting position.

Analysis

This exercise is separated into two movements for analysis: (1) movement to the knee-bend position and (2) return movement to starting position. NOTE: It is assumed that no movement will take place in the shoulder joint, shoulder girdle, wrists, hands, and back.

Movement to knee-bend position
  Hip
    Flexion
      Hip extensors (eccentric contraction)
        Gluteus maximus
        Semimembranosus
        Semitendinosus
        Biceps femoris

  Knee
    Flexion
      Knee extensors (eccentric contraction)
        Rectus femoris
        Vastus lateralis
        Vastus medialis
        Vastus intermedius
  Foot and ankle
    Dorsal flexion
      Plantar flexors (eccentric contraction)
        Gastrocnemius
        Soleus

Return movement to starting position
  Hip
    Extension
      Gluteus maximus
      Semimembranosus
      Semitendinosus
      Biceps femoris
  Knee
    Extension
      Rectus femoris
      Vastus lateralis
      Vastus medialis
      Vastus intermedius
  Foot and ankle
    Plantar flexion
      Gastrocnemius
      Soleus

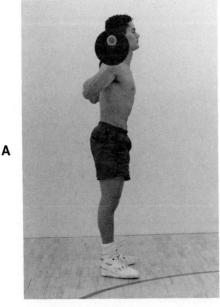

A

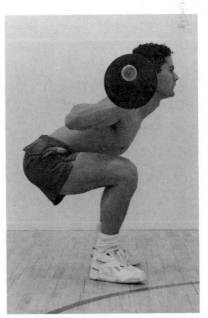

B

FIG. 11-3 ● Squat. **A**, Starting position; **B**, squatted position.

Dead lift

Description

The subject is in a standing position with the barbell held in the hands. He bends forward at the hip joints, keeping the arms, legs, and back straight, and touches the floor with the barbell. Then a movement to the standing position is made by extending the hips.

Analysis

This exercise is divided into two movements for analysis: (1) movement to bend over and to touch the barbell to the floor, and (2) return movement to standing position.

Movement to bend over and to touch barbell to floor

Wrist and hand
Flexion
Wrist and hand flexors
Flexor carpi radialis
Flexor carpi ulnaris
Palmaris longus
Flexor digitorum profundus
Flexor digitorum superficialis
Flexor pollicis longus

Trunk
Flexion
Trunk extensors (eccentric contraction)
Erector spinae
Quadratus lumborum

Hip
Flexion
Hip extensors (eccentric contraction)
Gluteus maximus
Semimembranosus
Semitendinosus
Biceps femoris

NOTE: Slight movement of the shoulder joint and girdle is not being analyzed.

Return movement to standing position

Wrist and hand
Flexion
Wrist and hand flexors
Flexor carpi radialis
Flexor carpi ulnaris
Palmaris longus
Flexor digitorum profundus
Flexor digitorum superficialis
Flexor pollicis longus

Trunk
Extension
Erector spinae (sacrospinalis)
Quadratus lumborum

Hip
Extension
Gluteus maximus
Semimembranosus
Semitendinosus
Biceps femoris

ISOMETRIC EXERCISES

An exercise technique called "isometrics" is a type of muscular activity in which there is contraction of muscle groups with little or no muscle shortening. Many magazine articles and books have been written about isometric exercises and their values. Although not as productive in terms of overall strength gains as isotonics, isometrics are an effective way to build and maintain muscular strength in a limited range of motion.

A few selected isometric exercises are analyzed muscularly to show how they are designed to develop specific muscle groups.

Abdominal contraction

Description

The subject contracts the muscles in the anterior abdominal region as strongly as possible with no movement of the trunk or hips. This exercise can be performed in sitting, standing, or supine positions. The longer the contraction in seconds, the more valuable the exercise will be, to a degree.

Analysis

Abdomen
Contraction
Rectus abdominis
External oblique abdominal
Internal oblique abdominal
Transversus abdominis

Shoulder pull
Description

In a standing or sitting position, the subject clasps the hands together in front of the chest and then attempts to pull them apart. This contraction is continued from 5 to 20 seconds.

Analysis

In this type of exercise there is little or no movement of the contracting muscles. In certain isometric exercises, contraction of the antagonistic muscles is as strong as the muscles attempting to produce the force for movement. The muscle groups contracting to produce a movement are designated the *agonists*. In the exercise just described, there are contractions of the antagonistic muscles of the wrist and hand, elbow, shoulder joint, and shoulder girdle. The strength of the contraction depends on the angle of pull and the leverage of the joint involved. Thus it is not the same at each point.

Attempted movements

Extension of wrist and hand—resisted by flexors of wrists and hand
  Agonist—wrist and hand extensors
  Antagonists—wrist and hand flexors
Extension of elbow joint—resisted by flexors of wrist, elbow, and hand
  Agonist—triceps brachii and anconeus
  Antagonist—biceps brachii, brachialis, brachioradialis
Abduction of shoulder joint—resisted by adductors of shoulder joint
  Agonist—deltoid and supraspinatus
  Antagonist—teres major, latissimus dorsi, pectoralis major
Adduction and depression of shoulder girdle—resisted by abductors
  Agonist—rhomboid and trapezius
  Antagonist—serratus anterior, pectoralis minor, trapezius (upper)

Isometric exercises vary in the number of muscles contracting, depending on the type of exercise and the joints at which there is attemped movement. The shoulder-pull exercise produces some contraction of antagonistic muscles at four sets of joints.

Leg lifter
Description

The subject sits on a bench or chair with the knees slightly bent and with one leg over the other. He attempts to raise the left leg while resisting it with the right leg.

Analysis*
Left leg—attempt upward movment
Foot and ankle
Dorsal flexion
  Tibialis anterior
  Extensor hallucis longus
  Extensor digitorum longus
  Peroneus tertius
Knee
Extension
  Quadriceps
    Rectus femoris
    Vastus lateralis
    Vastus medialis
    Vastus intermedius
Hip
Flexion
  Iliopsoas
  Rectus femoris
  Pectineus
  Sartorius
  Tensor fasciae latae
Right leg—resisting upward movment
Foot and ankle
Plantar flexion
  Gastrocnemius
  Soleus
Knee
Flexion
  Hamstrings
    Biceps femoris
    Semitendinosus
    Semimembranosus
Hip
Extension
  Gluteus maximus
  Biceps femoris
  Semitendinosus
  Semimembranosus

---

*When the legs are alternated, the muscles used will be the same muscles but in the other leg.

UNIVERSAL CONDITIONING MACHINE

The Universal conditioning machine* or similar machine by other manufacturers (Fig. 11-4) are used by professional, college, and many high-school athletes. Health clubs, YMCAs, YWCAs, fitness centers, and body gyms have these machines for use by their members. Many similar types of machines are available; these include Cybex Eagle Nautilus, Paramount, Olympus, and others.

All exercise machines come with a list of recommended exercises that can be done by the user. A few of the exercises for the Universal conditioning machine are analyzed in the following section. Fig. 11-5 is a daily record sheet that can be kept by the participant.

*Universal Athletics Sales Co., Inc., Fresno, Calif.

FIG. 11-4 • Universal conditioning machine with 16 separate stations.

Courtesy Universal Athletic Sales Co., Inc., Fresno, Calif.

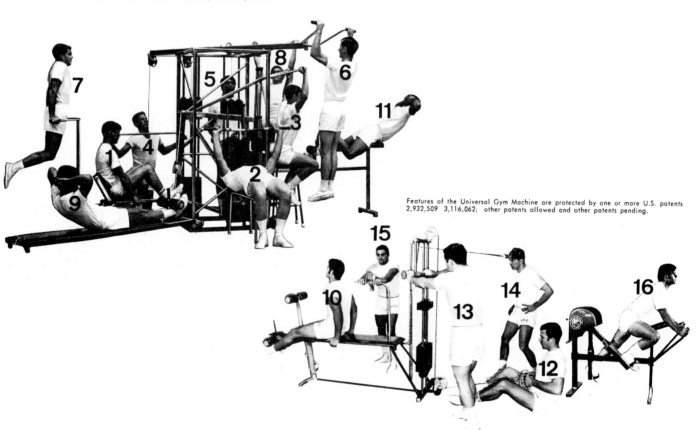

Features of the Universal Gym Machine are protected by one or more U.S. patents 2,932,509 3,116,062; other patents allowed and other patents pending.

1. Leg press
2. Chest press
3. Shoulder press
4. High lateral pull
5. Quad and dead lift station
6. Chinning station
7. Dipping station
8. Hip flexor
9. Abdominal conditioner
10. Thigh and knee machine
11. Back and hyperextension and swimmers' kick station
12. Wrist conditioner
13. Hand gripper station
14. Neck conditioner
15. Hand gripper station
16. Real-runner

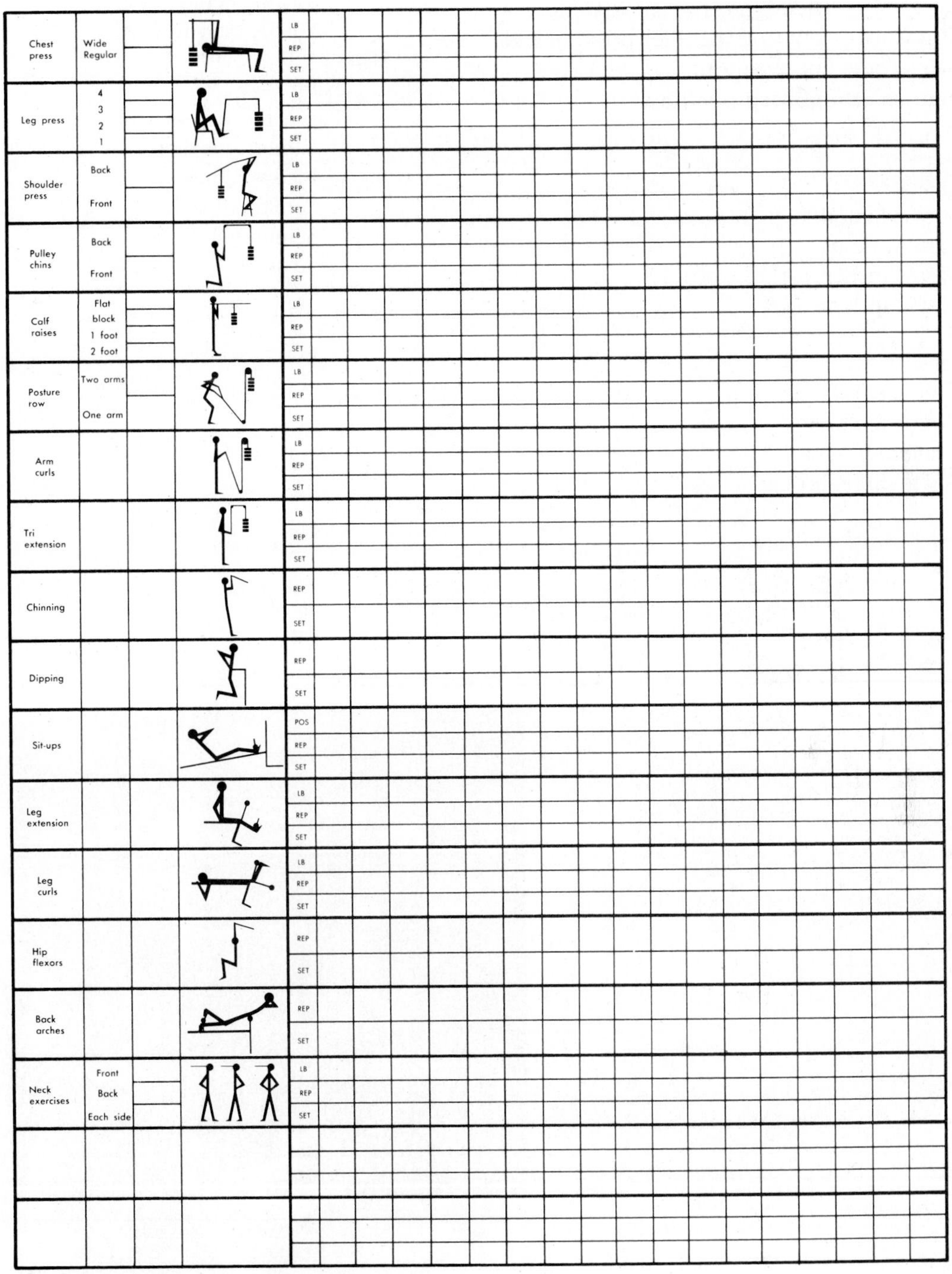

Exercise	Variation		(figure)	Measure																	
Chest press	Wide / Regular			LB / REP / SET																	
Leg press	4 / 3 / 2 / 1			LB / REP / SET																	
Shoulder press	Back / Front			LB / REP / SET																	
Pulley chins	Back / Front			LB / REP / SET																	
Calf raises	Flat block / 1 foot / 2 foot			LB / REP / SET																	
Posture row	Two arms / One arm			LB / REP / SET																	
Arm curls				LB / REP / SET																	
Tri extension				LB / REP / SET																	
Chinning				REP / SET																	
Dipping				REP / SET																	
Sit-ups				POS / REP / SET																	
Leg extension				LB / REP / SET																	
Leg curls				LB / REP / SET																	
Hip flexors				REP / SET																	
Back arches				REP / SET																	
Neck exercises	Front / Back / Each side			LB / REP / SET																	

FIG. 11-5 • Universal Spartacus daily record sheet.

Leg press FIG. 11-6

Description

The subject sits and presses until the knees are straight. Then he returns to the starting position.

Analysis

Leg press can be divided into two movements for analysis: (1) movement to straight-leg position and (2) return to standing position.

Movement to straight-leg position

Knee

Extension

Quadriceps

Rectus femoris

Vastus lateralis

Vastus medialis

Vastus intermedius

Hip

Extension

Gluteus maximus

Biceps femoris

Semitendinosus

Semimembranosus

Return to starting position

Knee

Flexion

Knee extensors (eccentric contraction)

Rectus femoris

Vastus lateralis

Vastus medialis

Vastus intermedius

Hip

Flexion

Hip extensors (eccentric contraction)

Gluteus maximus

Biceps femoris

Semitendinosus

Semimembranosus

FIG. 11-6 • Leg press.

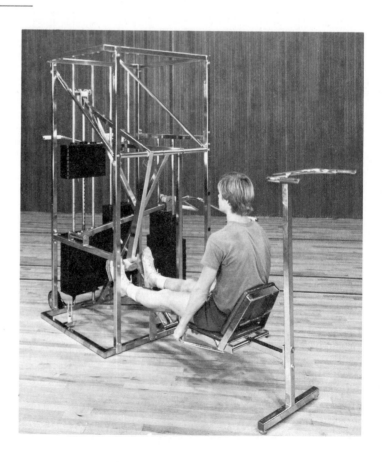

Triceps extension

Description

The subject stands in front of the machine with the arms flexed at the elbow, grasps the bar, and presses down until the arms are straight.

Analysis

This exercise can be divided into two movements for analysis: (1) movement to pressing arms down to straight-arm position, and (2) return movement to starting position.

Movement to straight-arm position
Wrist and hand
Flexion
  Wrist and hand flexors
    Flexor carpi radialis
    Flexor carpi ulnaris
    Palmaris longus
    Flexor digitorum profundus
    Flexor digitorum superficialis
    Flexor pollicis longus
Elbow joint
Extension
  Triceps brachii
  Anconeus
Shoulder joint
Extension
  Latissimus dorsi
  Teres major
  Posterior deltoid
  Pectoralis major (sternal head-lower fibers)
  Triceps brachii (long head)
Shoulder girdle
Adduction and depression
  Lower trapezius
  Pectoralis major

Return movement to starting position
Wrist and hand
Flexion
  Wrist and hand flexors
    Flexor carpi radialis
    Flexor carpi ulnaris
    Palmaris longus
    Flexor digitorum profundus
    Flexor digitorum superficialis
    Flexor pollicis longus
Elbow joint
Flexion
  Elbow extensors (eccentric contraction)
    Triceps brachii
    Anconeus
Shoulder joint
Flexion
  Shoulder joint extensors (eccentric contraction)
    Latissimus dorsi
    Teres major
    Posterior deltoid
    Pectoralis major (sternal head-lower fibers)
    Triceps brachii (long head)
Shoulder girdle
Abduction
  Shoulder joint abductors (eccentric contraction)
    Lower trapezius
    Pectoralis major

Chest press (bench press)

Description

The subject lies on the exercise bench in the supine position, grasps the apparatus hand holds, and presses the weight upward through the full range of arm and shoulder movement. Then the weight is lowered to the starting position (see Fig. 11-4).

Analysis

The chest press can be divided into two movements for analysis: (1) upward movement to length of arms, and (2) return movement to the starting position.

Movement to upward position

Wrist and hand

Flexion

Wrist and hand flexors

Flexor carpi radialis

Flexor carpi ulnaris

Palmaris longus

Flexor digitorum profundus

Flexor digitorum superficialis

Flexor pollicis longus

Elbow joint

Extension

Triceps brachii

Anconeus

Shoulder joint

Flexion and horizontal adduction

Pectoralis major

Anterior deltoid

Coracobrachialis

Biceps brachii

Shoulder girdle

Abduction

Serratus anterior

Pectoralis minor

Return movement to starting position

Wrist and hand

Flexion

Wrist and hand flexors

Flexor carpi radialis

Flexor carpi ulnaris

Palmaris longus

Flexor digitorum profundus

Flexor digitorum superficialis

Flexor pollicis longus

Elbow joint

Flexion

Elbow extensors (eccentric contraction)

Triceps brachii

Anconeus

Shoulder joint

Extension and horizontal abduction

Shoulder joint flexors and horizontal adductors (eccentric contraction)

Pectoralis major

Anterior deltoid

Coracobrachialis

Biceps brachii

Shoulder girdle

Adduction and depression

Shoulder girdle abductors (eccentric contraction)

Serratus anterior

Pectoralis minor

Modern exercise machines

With the physical revolution of the past several decades has come the development of many new exercise machines. Some machines are engineered to have a constant resistance throughout the range of movement. A number of companies have developed individual machines for exercising many of the large muscle groups of the human body: quadriceps, hamstrings, abdominals, neck, pectoral, and other muscle groups.

Hip sled   FIG. 11-7

Description

The subject lies in a supine position on the floor with the knees and hips flexed in a position close to the chest. The feet are placed on the apparatus plate. The plate is moved upward until the knees and hips are completely extended. Then the subject returns to the starting position.

Analysis

This exercise is divided into two movements for analysis: (1) movement upward to high position, and (2) return movement to the starting position.

Movement upward to high position

  Foot and ankle

    Plantar flexion

      Gastrocnemius

      Soleus

  Knee

    Extension

      Quadriceps

      Rectus femoris

      Vastus medialis

      Vastus intermedius

      Vastus lateralis

  Hip

    Extension

      Biceps femoris

      Semimembranosus

      Semitendinosus

      Gluteus maximus

Return movement to starting position

  Foot and ankle

    Dorsal flexion

      Plantar flexors (eccentric contraction)

        Gastrocnemius

        Soleus

  Knee

    Flexion

      Knee extensors (eccentric contraction)

        Rectus femoris

        Vastus medialis

        Vastus intermedius

        Vastus lateralis

  Hip

    Flexion

      Hip extensors (eccentric contraction)

        Biceps femoris

        Semimembranosus

        Semitendinosus

        Gluteus maximus

FIG. 11-7 • Hip sled (hip and leg press.)
A, Starting position; **B**, high position.

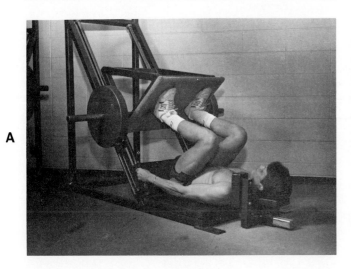
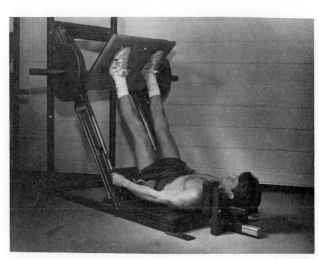

A

B

Rowing exercise FIG. 11-8

Description

The subject sits on a movable seat with the knees and hips flexed close to the chest. The arms are reaching forward (see Fig. 11-8) to grasp a horizontal bar. The legs are extended forcibly as the arms are pulled toward the chest. Then the legs and arms are returned to the starting position.

Analysis

This exercise is divided into two movements for analysis: (1) movement to extend the legs forward and arms pulled toward the chest, and (2) return movement to the starting position.

Movement to extend the legs forward and arms pulled toward the chest

Foot and ankle
  Plantar flexion
    Gastrocnemius
    Soleus

Knee
  Extension
    Rectus femoris
    Vastus intermedius
    Vastus lateralis
    Vastus medialis

Hip
  Extension
    Gluteus maximus
    Biceps femoris
    Semimembranosus
    Semitendinosus

Trunk
  Extension
    Erector spinae

Shoulder girdle
  Adduction and depression
    Trapezius (lower)
    Rhomboid
    Pectoralis minor

Shoulder joint
  Extension
    Latissimus dorsi
    Teres major
    Posterior deltoid
    Teres minor
    Infraspinatus

Elbow joint
  Flexion
    Biceps brachii
    Brachialis
    Brachioradialis

Wrist and hand
  Flexion
    Flexor carpi radialis
    Flexor carpi ulnaris
    Palmaris longus
    Flexor digitorum profundus
    Flexor digitorum superficialis
    Flexor pollicis longus

Return to the starting position

Foot and ankle
  Dorsal flexion
    Tibial anterior
    Extensor hallucis longus
    Extensor digitorum longus
    Peroneus tertius

Knee
  Extension
    Biceps femoris
    Semitendinosus
    Semimembranosus

Hip
  Flexion
    Iliopsoas
    Rectus femoris
    Pectineus

Trunk
  Flexion
    Rectus abdominus
    Internal oblique abdominal
    External oblique abdominal

Shoulder girdle
  Abduction and elevation
    Shoulder girdle adductors and depressors (eccentric contraction)

Shoulder joint
  Flexion
    Shoulder joint extensors (eccentric contraction)

Elbow joint
  Extension
    Elbow joint flexors (eccentric contraction)

Wrist and hand
  Flexion
    Wrist and hand flexors

FIG. 11-8 • Rowing exercise machine **A,** Starting position; **B,** movement.

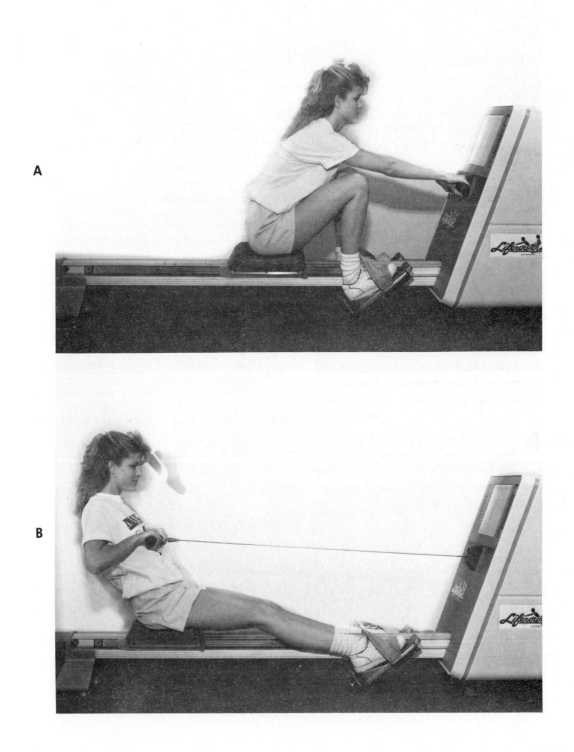

Worksheet exercises

As an aid to learning, for in-class and out-of-class assignments, or for testing, take any exercise from the Universal Spartacus daily record sheet.

1. Using the techniques taught in this chapter and Chapter 6, analyze the joint movements and muscles used in the exercise.

Laboratory and review exercises

1. Obtain, describe, and completely analyze five conditioning exercises.
2. Collect, analyze, and evaluate exercises that are found in newspapers and magazines or are observed on television.
3. Prepare a set of exercises that will ensure development of all large muscle groups in the body.
4. Select exercises from exercise books for analysis.
5. Bring to class other typical exercises for members to analyze.
6. Analyze the conditioning exercises given by your physical education teachers or varsity coaches.
7. Observe children using playground equipment. Analyze muscularly the activities they are performing.
8. Visit the room on your campus where the heavy apparatus (Universal or similar machine) is located. Analyze exercises that can be done with the machine.
9. Consider a sport (basketball or any other sport) and develop exercises applying the overload principle that would develop all the large muscle groups used in the sport.

NOTE: Manufacturers of all types of exercise apparatus have a complete list of exercises that can be performed with their machines. Secure a copy of recommended exercises and muscularly analyze each exercise.

References

Altug Z, Hoffman JL, Martin JL: Manual of clinical exercise testing, prescription and rehabilitation, Norwalk, Conn, 1993, Appleton & Lange.

Andrews JR, Harrelson GL: Physical rehabilitation of the injured athlete, Philadelphia, 1991, Saunders.

Baitch SP: Aerobic dance injuries, a biomechanical approach, Journal of Physcial Education, Recreation and Dance 58:57, May-June 1987.

Bouche J: Three essential lifts for high school players, Scholastic Coach 56:42, April 1987.

Brzycki M: R$_x$ for a safe productive strength program, Scholastic Coach 57:70, September 1987.

Epley B: Getting elementary muscles, Coach and Athlete 44:60, November-December 1981.

Fahey TD: Athletic training: principles and practices, Mountain View, Ca, 1986, Mayfield.

Logan GA, McKinney WC: Anatomic kinesiology, ed. 3, Dubuque, Ia, 1982, Brown.

Matheson O, et al: Stress fractures in athletes, American Journal of Sports Medicine 15:46, January-February 1987.

Minton S: Dance dynamics avoiding dance injuries (symposium), Journal of Physical Education, Recreation and Dance 58:29, May-June 1987.

Northrip JW, Logan GA, McKinney WC: Analysis of sport motion: anatomic and biomechanic perspectives, ed 3, Dubuque, Ia, 1983, Brown.

Prentice WE: Rehabilitation techniques in sports medicine, St. Louis, 1990, Mosby.

Schlitz J: The athlete's daily dozen stretches, Athletic Journal 66:20, November 1985.

Todd J: Strength training for female athletes, Journal of Physical Education, Recreation and Dance, 56:38, August 1985.

Torg JS, Vegso JJ, Torg E: Rehabilitation of athletic injuries: an atlas of therapeutic exercise, Chicago, 1987, Year Book.

Wirhed R: Athletic ability and the anatomy of motion, London, 1984, Wolfe.

Some factors affecting motion and movement

12

Objectives

• To know and understand how knowledge of levers can help improve physical performance.

• To know and understand how knowledge of lever arm lengths and angles of pull can help improve physical performance.

• To know and understand how knowledge of Newton's laws of motion can help improve physical performance.

• To know and understand how knowledge of balance, equilibrium, and stability can help improve physical performance.

• To know and understand how knowledge of force and momentum can help improve physical performance.

Many students in kinesiology classes have some knowledge, from a college or high school physics or physical science course, of the physical laws that affect motion. They need to review these facts and principles as they learn to apply them to motion in the human body.

A brief discussion of some of these principles follows.

Levers

It is difficult for a person to visualize his body as a system of levers. The topic may seem academic to some, but this is far from true. A person moves through the use of his system of levers. The anatomical levers of the body cannot be changed, but when properly understood, the system can be more efficiently used to maximize the muscular efforts of the body.

A lever is defined as a rigid bar that turns about an *axis* of rotation or a fulcrum. The axis is the point of rotation about which the lever moves.

The lever rotates about the axis as a result of *force* (sometimes referred to as effort, *E*) being applied to it to cause its movement against a *resistance* or weight. In the body, the bones represent the bars, the joints are the axes, and the muscles contract to apply the force. The amount of resistance can vary from maximal to minimal. In fact, the bones themselves or weight of the body segment may be the only resistance applied. All lever systems have each of these three components in one of three possible arrangements.

The arrangement or location of these three points in relation to one another determine the type of lever and for which kind of motion it is best suited. These points are the axis, the point of force application (usually the muscle insertion), and the point of resistance application (sometimes the center of gravity of the lever and sometimes the location of an external resistance). When the axis *(A)* is placed between the force *(F)* and the resistance *(R)*, a first-class lever is produced (Figs. 12-1 and 12-2). In second-class levers the resistance is between the axis and the force (Figs. 12-1 and 12-3). If the force is placed between the axis and the resistance, a third-class lever is created (Figs. 12-1 and 12-4).

First-class levers

Typical examples of a first-class lever are the crowbar, seesaw, and elbow extension. An example of this type of lever in the body is seen with the triceps applying the force to the olecranon *(F)* in extending the nonsupported forearm *(R)* at the elbow *(A)*. Other examples of this type of lever may be seen in the body when the agonist and antagonist muscle groups on either side of a joint axis are contracting simultaneously with the agonist producing force while the antagonist supplies the resistance. A first-class lever (Fig. 12-2) is designed basically to produce balanced movements when the axis is midway between the force and the resistance (e.g., seesaw). When the axis is close to the force, the lever produces speed and range of motion (e.g., triceps in elbow extension). When the axis is close to the resistance, the lever produces force motion (e.g., crowbar).

In applying the principle of levers to the body it is important to remember that the force is applied where the muscle inserts in the bone and not in the belly of the muscle. For example, in elbow extension with the shoulder fully flexed and the arm beside the ear, the triceps applies the force to the olecranon of the ulna behind the axis of the elbow joint. As the applied force exceeds the amount of forearm resistance, the elbow extends.

The type of lever may be changed for a given joint and muscle, depending on whether the body segment is in contact with a surface such as a floor or wall. For example, we have demonstrated the triceps in elbow extension being a first-class lever with the hand free in space where the arm is pushed upward away from the body. By placing the hand in contact with the floor, as in performing a push-up to push the body away from the floor, the same muscle action at this joint now changes the lever to second class because the axis is at the hand and the resistance is the body weight at the elbow joint.

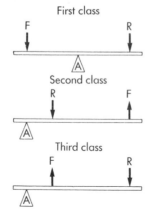

FIG. 12-1 • Classification of levers.

Modified from Hall SJ: Basic biomechanics, St. Louis, 1991, Mosby.

FIG. 12-2 • **A** and **B**, First-class levers.

A modified from Booher JM, Thibodeau GA: Athletic injury assessment, ed 2, St. Louis, 1989, Mosby; **B** modified from Hall SJ, Basic biomechanics, St. Louis, 1991, Mosby.

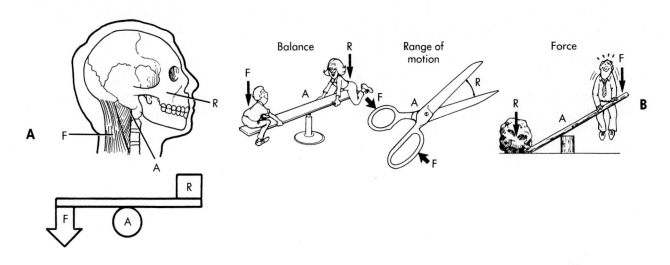

Second-class levers

A second-class lever (Fig. 12-3) is designed to produce force movements, since a large resistance can be moved by a relatively small force. An example of a second-class lever is a wheelbarrow. Besides the example given above of the triceps extending the elbow in a push-up another similar example of a second-class lever in the body is plantar flexion of the foot to raise the body up on the toes. The ball *(A)* of the foot serves as the axis of rotation as the ankle plantar flexors apply force to the calcaneus *(F)* to lift the resistance of the body at the tibial articulation *(R)* with the foot. There are relatively few occurrences of second-class levers in the body.

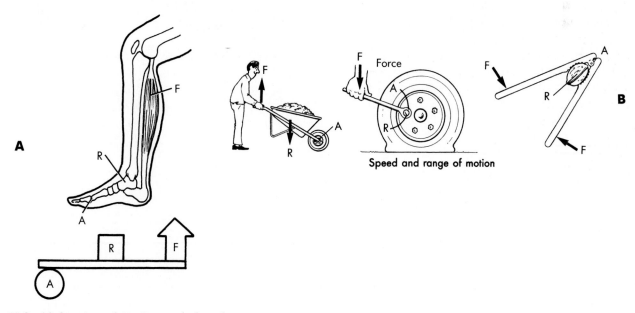

FIG. 12-3 • **A** and **B**, Second-class levers.

A modified from Booher JM, Thibodeau GA: Athletic injury assessment, ed 2, St Louis, 1989, Mosby; **B** modified from Hall SJ: Basic biomechanics, St. Louis, 1991, Mosby.

Third-class levers

Third-class levers (Fig. 12-4), with the force being applied between the axis and the resistance, are designed to produce speed and range-of-motion movements. Most of the levers in the human body are of this type, which require a great deal of force to move even a small resistance. Examples include a screen door operated by a short spring and application of lifting force to a shovel handle with the lower hand while the upper hand on the shovel handle serves as the axis of rotation. The biceps brachii is a typical example in the body. Using the elbow joint *(A)* as the axis, the biceps brachii applies force at its insertion on the radial tuberosity *(F)* to rotate the forearm up, with its center of gravity *(R)* serving as the point of resistance application.

The brachialis is an example of true third-class leverage. It pulls on the ulna just below the elbow, and since the ulna cannot rotate, the pull is direct and true. The biceps brachii, on the other hand, supinates the forearm as it flexes, so that the third-class leverage applies to flexion only.

Other examples include the hamstrings contracting to flex the leg at the knee while in a standing position and using the iliopsoas to flex the thigh at the hip.

FIG. 12-4 • **A** and **B**, Third-class levers.

A modified from Booher JM, Thibodeau GA: Athletic injury assessment, ed 2, St. Louis, 1989, Mosby; **B** modified from Hall SJ: Basic biomechanics, St. Louis, 1991, Mosby.

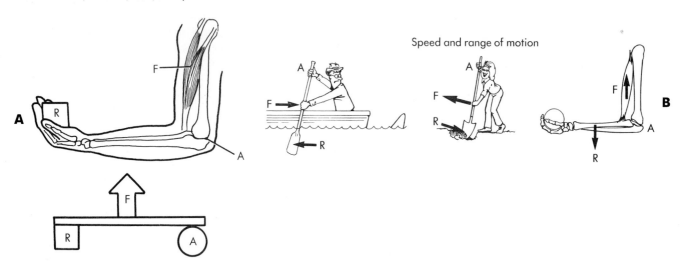

Factors in use of anatomical levers

Our anatomical leverage system can be used to gain a mechanical advantage that will improve simple or complex physical movements. Some individuals unconsciously develop habits of using human levers properly, but frequently this is not true.

Length of lever arms

In discussing the application of levers, it is necessary to understand the length relationship between the two lever arms. The *resistance arm* is the distance between the axis and the point of resistance application, whereas the distance between the axis and the point of force application is known as the *force arm*. There is an inverse relationship between force and the force arm just as there is between resistance and the resistance arm. The longer the force arm, the less force required to move the lever if the resistance and resistance arm remain constant. In addition, if the force and force arm remain constant, a greater resistance may be moved by shortening the resistance arm.

Also, there is a proportional relationship between the force components and the resistance components. That is, for movement to occur when either of the resistance components increase, there must be an increase in one or both of the force components. Even slight variations in the location of the force and resistance are important in determining the effective force of the muscle. This point can be illustrated in the following simple formula, using the biceps brachii muscle in each example.

$$\underset{\text{(Force)}}{F} \times \underset{\substack{\text{(Force} \\ \text{arm)}}}{FA} = \underset{\text{(Resistance)}}{R} \times \underset{\substack{\text{(Resistance} \\ \text{arm)}}}{RA}$$

Initial example

$$F \times 2 \text{ inches} = 10 \text{ pounds} \times 9 \text{ inches}$$
$$2 F = 90 \text{ pounds}$$
$$F = 45 \text{ pounds}$$

Example A
Change the insertion (FA) 1 inch:

$$F \times 3 \text{ inches} = 10 \text{ pounds} \times 9 \text{ inches}$$
$$3 F = 90 \text{ pounds}$$
$$F = 30 \text{ pounds}$$

A change of 1 inch in the insertion can make a considerable difference in the force necessary to move the lever.

Example B
Change the point of resistance application (RA) 1 inch:

$$F \times 2 \text{ inches} = 10 \text{ pounds} \times 8 \text{ inches}$$
$$2 F = 80 \text{ pounds}$$
$$F = 40 \text{ pounds}$$

Shortening the resistance arm can decrease the amount of force necessary to move the lever.

Example C
Change the amount of resistance (R) 1 pound:

$$F \times 2 \text{ inches} = 9 \text{ pounds} \times 9 \text{ inches}$$
$$2 F = 81 \text{ pounds}$$
$$F = 40.5 \text{ pounds}$$

Obviously decreasing the amount of resistance can decrease the amount of force needed to move the lever.

The system of leverage in the human body is built for speed and range of movement at the expense of force. Short force arms and long resistance arms require great muscular strength to produce movement. In the forearm, the attachments of the biceps and triceps muscles clearly illustrate this point, since the force arm of the biceps is 1 to 2 inches and that of the triceps less than 1 inch. Many other similar examples are found all over the body. From a practical point of view, this means that the muscular system should be strong to supply the necessary force for body movements, especially in strenuous sports activities.

When we speak of human leverage in relation to sport skills, we are generally referring to several levers. For example, in throwing a ball there are levers at the shoulder, elbow, and wrist joints.

In fact, it can be said that there is one long lever from the feet to the hand.

The longer the lever, the more effective it is in imparting velocity. A tennis player can hit a tennis ball harder with a straight-arm drive than with a bent elbow because the lever (including the racket) is longer and moves at a faster speed.

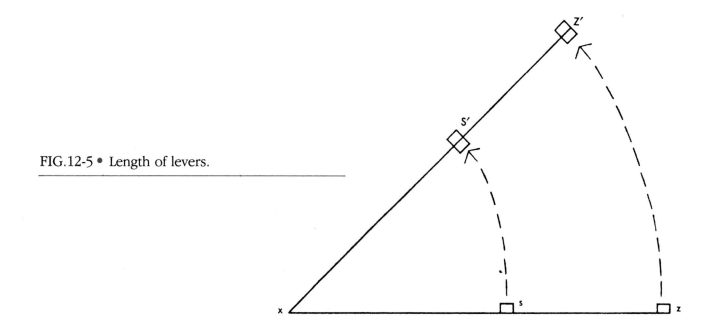

FIG.12-5 • Length of levers.

Fig. 12-5 indicates that a longer lever (Z') travels faster than a shorter lever (S') in traveling the same number of degrees. In sports activities in which it is possible to increase the length of a lever with a racket or bat, the same principle applies.

In baseball, hockey, golf, field hockey, and other sports, long levers similarly produce more linear force and thus better performance. For quickness of movement, it is sometimes desirable to have a short lever arm, such as when a baseball catcher brings his hand back to his ear to secure a quick throw or when a sprinter shortens his knee lever through flexion so much that he almost catches his spikes in his gluteal muscles.

Angle of pull

Another factor of considerable importance in using the leverage system is the *angle of pull* of the muscles on the bone. The angle of pull may be defined as the angle between the muscle insertion and the bone on which it inserts. Joint movements and insertion angles involve mostly small angles of pull. The angle increases as the bone moves away from its anatomical position through the contraction of the local muscle group. This range of movement depends on the type of joint and bony structure.

Most muscles work at a small angle of pull, generally less than 50 degrees. At 90 degrees, all of the force of a muscle is rotary force. That is, all of the force is being used to rotate the lever about its axis. At all other degrees of the angle of pull, there are two components of force operating. One is the same *rotary component* that is continuing, although with less force, to rotate the lever about its axis. The second force component is either a *stabilizing component* or a *dislocating component*, depending on whether the angle of pull is less than or greater than 90 degrees. If the angle is less than 90 degrees, the force is a dislocating force because it is pulling the bone away from the joint center. If the angle is greater than 90 degrees, the force is stabilizing due to its pulling the bone toward the center of the joint (Fig.12-6).

In some activities it is desirable to have a person begin a movement when the angle of pull is at 90 degrees. Many boys and girls are unable to do a chin-up (pull-up) unless they start with the elbow in a position to allow the elbow flexor muscle group to approximate a 90-degree angle with the forearm.

This angle makes the chin-up easier because of the more advantageous angle of pull. The application of this fact can compensate for lack of sufficient strength. In its range of motion, a muscle pulls a lever through a range characteristic of itself, but in approaching and going beyond 90 degrees, it is most effective. An increase in strength is the only solution for muscles that operate at disadvantageous angles of pull and require a greater force to operate efficiently.

FIG. 12-6 • **A** to **C**, Components of force due to
the angle of pull.

Modified from Hall SJ: *Basic biomechanics,* St. Louis, 1991, Mosby.

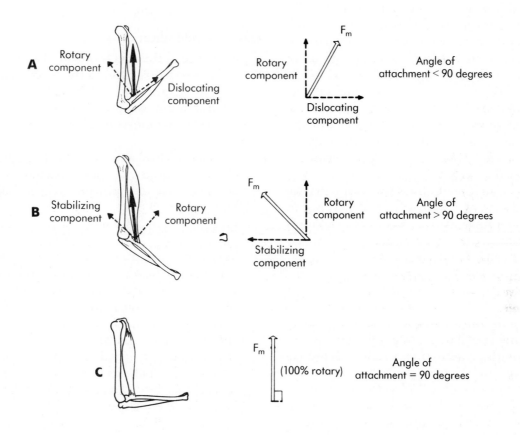

Laws of motion and physical activities

Motion is fundamental in physical education and sports activity. Body motion is generally produced or at least started by some action of the muscular system. Motion cannot occur without a force, and the muscular system is the source of force in the human body. Thus development of the muscular system is indispensable to movement.

Basically, there are two types of motion: *linear motion* and *angular motion*. Linear motion, also referred to as translatory motion, is motion along a line. If the motion is along a straight line, it is rectilinear motion, whereas motion along a curved line is known as curvilinear motion. Angular motion involves rotation around an axis. In the human body the axis of rotation is provided by the various joints. In a sense, these two types of motion are related, since angular motion of the joints can produce the linear motion of walking.

For example, in many sports activities the cumulative angular motion of the joints of the body imparts linear motion to a thrown object (ball, shot) or to an object struck with an instrument (bat, racket).

A brief review of Newton's laws of motion will indicate the many applications of these laws to physical education activities and sports. Newton's laws explain all the characteristics of motion and are fundamental to understanding human movement.

Law of inertia

A body in motion tends to remain in motion at the same speed in a straight line; a body at rest tends to remain at rest unless acted on by a force.

Inertia may be described as the resistance to action or change. In terms of human movement, inertia refers to resistance to acceleration or deceleration. Inertia is the tendency for the current state of motion to be maintained, regardless of whether the body segment is moving at a particular velocity or is motionless.

Muscles produce the force necessary to start motion, stop motion, accelerate motion, decelerate motion, or change the direction of motion. Put another way, inertia is the reluctance to change status; only force can do it. Numerous examples of this law are found in physical education activities. A sprinter in his starting blocks must apply considerable force to overcome his resting inertia. A runner on an indoor track must apply consid-

erable force to overcome moving inertia and stop before hitting the wall. Balls and other objects that are thrown or struck require force to stop them. Starting, stopping, and changing direction—a part of many physical activities—provide many other examples of the law of inertia applied to body motion.

Since force is required to change inertia, it is obvious that any activity that is carried out at a steady pace in a consistent direction will conserve energy, and any irregularly paced or directed activity will be very costly to energy reserves. This explains in part why activities such as handball and basketball are so much more fatiguing than jogging or dancing.

Law of acceleration

A change in the acceleration of a body occurs in the same direction as the force that caused it. The change in acceleration is directly proportional to the force causing it and inversely proportional to the mass of the body.

Acceleration may be defined as the rate of change in velocity. To attain speed in moving the body, a strong muscular force is generally necessary (*weight*). Weight or, more technically, "mass" (gravity) affects the speed and acceleration in physical movements. It requires a much greater force from the muscles to accelerate a 230-pound man than it does a 130-pound man to the same running speed. Also, it is possible to accelerate a baseball faster than a shot because of the difference in weight. The force required to run at half speed is less than the force required to run at top speed. To impart speed to a ball or an object, it is necessary to rapidly accelerate the part of the body holding the object. Football, basketball, track, and field hockey are a few sports that demand speed and acceleration.

Law of reaction

For every action there is an opposite and equal reaction.

As we place force on a supporting surface by walking over it, the surface provides an equal resistance back in the opposite direction to the soles of our feet. It is easier to run on a hard track than on a sandy beach because of the difference in the reactions of the two surfaces. The track resists the runner's propulsion force, and the reaction drives the runner ahead. The sand dissipates the runner's force, and the reaction force is correspondingly reduced with the apparent loss in forward force and speed. A sprinter applies a force in excess of 300 pounds on his starting blocks, which resist with an equal force. When a body is in flight, as it is in jumping, movement of one part of the body produces a reaction in another part. This occurs because there is no resistive surface to supply a reaction force.

Balance, equilibrium, and stability

Balance is the ability to control equilibrium, either static or dynamic. In relation to human movement, *equilibrium* refers to a state of zero acceleration where there is no change in the speed or direction of the body. Equilibrium may be either static or dynamic. If the body is at rest or completely motionless, it is in *static equilibrium. Dynamic equilibrium* occurs when all of the applied and inertial forces acting on the moving body are in balance, resulting in movement with unchanging speed or direction. For us to control equilibrium and hence achieve balance, we need to maximize *stability*. Stability is the resistance to a change in the body's acceleration or more appropriately the resistance to a disturbance of the body's equilibrium. Stability may be enhanced by determining the body's *center of gravity* and changing it appropriately. The center of gravity is the point at which all of body's mass and weight is equally balanced or equally distributed in all directions.

Balance is important for the resting body, as well as for the moving body. Generally, balance is to be desired, but there are circumstances in which movement is improved when the body tends to be unbalanced. Following are certain general factors that apply toward enhancing equilibrium, maximizing stability, and ultimately achieving balance:

1. A person has balance when the center of gravity falls within the base of support.
2. A person has balance in the direct proportion to the size of the base. The larger the base of support, the more balance.
3. A person has balance depending on the weight (mass). The greater the weight, the more balance.
4. A person has balance, depending on the height of the center of gravity. The lower the center of gravity, the more balance.
5. A person has balance, depending on where the center of gravity is in relation to the base of support. The balance is less if the center of gravity is near the edge of the base. However, when anticipating an oncoming force, stability may be improved by placing the center of gravity nearer the side of the base of support expected to receive the force.
6. In anticipation of an oncoming force, stability may be increased by enlarging the size of the base of support in the direction of the anticipated force.
7. Equilibrium may be enhanced by increasing the friction between the body and the surfaces it contacts.
8. Rotation about an axis aids balance. A moving bike is easier to balance than a stationary bike.
9. Kinesthetic physiological functions contribute to balance. The semicircular canals of the inner ear, vision, touch (pressure), and kinesthetic sense all provide balance information to the performer. Balance and its components of equilibrium and stability are essential in all movements. They are all affected by the constant force of gravity as well as by inertia. Walking has been described as an activity in which a person throws the body in and out of balance with each step. In rapid running movements in which moving inertia is high, the individual has to lower the center of gravity to maintain balance when stopping or changing direction. On the other hand, jumping activities attempt to raise the center of gravity as high as possible.

Force

Muscles are the main source of force that produces or changes movement of a body segment, the entire body, or some object thrown, struck, or stopped. Strong muscles are able to produce more force than weak muscles. This refers to both maximum and sustained exertion over a period of time.

Forces either push or pull on an object in an attempt to affect motion or shape. Force is the product of mass times acceleration. *Mass* is the amount of matter in a body. For our purposes we can let weight serve as the mass. The weight of a body segment or the entire body times the speed of acceleration determines the force. Obviously in football this is very important. Yet it is just as important in other activities that use only a part of the human body. When one throws a ball, the force applied to the ball is equal to the weight of the arm times the speed of acceleration of the arm. Also, as previously discussed, the leverage factor is important.

The quantity of motion or, more scientifically stated, the *momentum*, which is equal to mass times velocity, is important in skill activities. The greater the momentum, the greater the resistance to change in the inertia or state of motion.

It is not necessary to apply maximum force and thus increase the momentum of a ball or object being struck in all situations. In skillful performance, regulation of the amount of force is necessary. Judgment as to the amount of force required to throw a softball a given distance, hit a golf ball 200 yards, or hit a tennis ball across the net and into the court is important.

In activities involving movement of various joints, as in throwing a ball or putting a shot, there should be a summation of forces from the beginning of movement in the lower segment of the body to the twisting of the trunk and movement at the shoulder, elbow, and wrist joints. The speed at which a golf club strikes the ball is the result of a summation of forces of the trunk, shoulders, arms, and wrists. Shot-putting and discus and javelin throwing are other good examples that show that summation of forces is essential.

Throwing

In the performance of various sport skills, many applications of the laws of leverage, motion, and balance may be found. A skill common to many activities is throwing. The object thrown may be some type of ball, but it is frequently an object of another size or shape, such as a rock, beanbag, Frisbee, discus, or javelin. A brief analysis of some of the basic mechanical principles involved in the skill of throwing will help to indicate the importance of understanding the applications of these principles. Many activities involve these and sometimes other mechanical principles. Motion is basic to throwing when the angular motion (p. 198) of the levers (bones) of the body (trunk, shoulder, elbow, and wrist) is used to give linear motion to the ball when it is released.

Newton's laws of motion apply in throwing because the individual's inertia and the ball's inertia (p. 198) must be overcome by the application of force. The muscles of the body provide the force to move the body parts and the ball held in the hand. The *law of acceleration* (Newton's second law) comes into operation with the muscular force necessary to accelerate the arm, wrist,

and hand. The greater the force (mass times acceleration) that a person can produce, the faster the arm will move, and thus the greater the speed that will be imparted to the ball. The reaction of the feet against the surface on which the subject stands indicates the application of the *law of reaction*.

The leverage factor is very important in throwing a ball or object. The longer the lever, the greater the speed that can be imparted to the ball. For all practical purposes, the body from the feet to the fingers can be considered as one long lever. The longer the lever, either from natural body length or from the movements of the body to the extended backward position (as in throwing a softball, with extension of the shoulder and the elbow joints), the greater will be the arc through which it accelerates and thus the greater the speed imparted to the thrown object.

In certain circumstances, when the ball is to be thrown only a short distance, as in baseball when it is thrown by the catcher to the bases, the short lever would be advantageous because it is faster. Balance or equilibrium is a factor in throwing when the body is rotated to the rear in the beginning of the throw. This motion moves the body nearly out of balance to the rear, and then balance changes again in the body with the forward movement. Balance is again established with the follow-through when the feet are spread and the knees and trunk are flexed to lower the center of gravity.

Summary

The preceding discussion has been a brief overview of some of the factors affecting motion. Analysis of human motion in light of the laws of physics poses a problem: How comprehensive is the analysis to be? It can become very complex, particularly when body motion is combined with the manipulation of an object in the hand involved in throwing, kicking, striking, or catching.

These factors become involved when an analysis is attempted of the activities common to our physical education program—football, baseball, basketball, track and field, field hockey, and swimming, to mention a few. However, a physical educator who is to have a complete view of which factors control human movement must have a working knowledge of both the physiological and the biomechanical principles of kinesiology.

It is beyond the scope of this book to make a detailed analysis of other activities. Some sources that consider these problems in detail are listed in the references.

Worksheet exercises

1. Special projects and class reports by individual or small groups of students on the mechanical analysis of all the skills involved in the following:
   a. Basketball
   b. Baseball
   c. Dancing
   d. Diving
   e. Football
   f. Field Hockey
   g. Golf
   h. Gymnastics
   i. Soccer
   j. Swimming
   k. Tennis
   l. Wrestling
2. Term projects and special class reports by individual or small groups of students about the following factors in motion:
   a. Balance
   b. Force
   c. Gravity
   d. Motion
   e. Leverage
   f. Projectiles
   g. Friction
   h. Buoyancy
   i. Aerodynamics
   j. Hydrodynamics
   k. Restitution
   l. Spin
   m. Rebound angle
   n. Momentum
   o. Center of gravity
   p. Equilibrium
   q. Stability
   r. Base of support
   s. Inertia
3. Demonstrations, term projects, or special reports by individual or small groups of students on the following activities:
   a. Lifting
   b. Throwing
   c. Standing
   d. Walking
   e. Running
   f. Jumping
   g. Falling
   h. Sitting
   i. Pushing and pulling
   j. Striking

References

Adrian MJ, Cooper JM: The biomechanics of human movement, Indianapolis, Ind, 1989, Benchmark Press.

American Academy of Orthopaedic Surgeons: Athletic training and sports medicine, ed 2, Park Ridge, Ill, 1991, American Academy of Orthopaedic Surgeons.

Barham JN: Mechanical kinesiology, St. Louis, 1978, Mosby.

Broer MR: An introduction to kinesiology, Englewood Cliffs, NJ, 1968, Prentice-Hall.

Broer MR, Zernicke RF: Efficiency of human movement, ed 3, Philadelphia, 1979, Saunders.

Bunn JW: Scientific principles of coaching, ed 2, Englewood Cliffs, NJ, 1972, Prentice-Hall.

Cooper JM, Adrian M, Glassow RB: Kinesiology, ed 5, St. Louis, 1982, Mosby.

Donatelli R, Wolf SL: The biomechanics of the foot and ankle, Philadelphia, 1990, Davis.

Exer-Genie instruction manual, Fullerton, Calif, 1966, Exer-Genie.

Hall SJ: Basic biomechanics, St. Louis, 1991, Mosby.

Hinson M: Kinesiology, ed 2, Dubuque, Ia, 1981, Brown.

Kegerreis S, Jenkins WL, Malone TR: Throwing injuries, Sports Injury Management 2:4, Baltimore, 1989, Williiams & Wilkins.

Kelley DL: Kinesiology: fundamentals of motion description, Englewood Cliffs, NJ, 1971, Prentice-Hall.

Kreighbaum E, Barthels KM: Biomechanics: a qualitative approach for studying human movement, ed. 3, New York, 1990, Macmillan.

Logan GA, McKinney WC: Anatomic kinesiology, ed 3, Dubuque, Ia, 1982, William.

Nordin M, Frankel VH: Basic biomechanics of the musculoskeletal system, ed 2, Philadelphia, 1989, Lea & Febiger.

Norkin CC, Levangie PK: Joint structure and function: a comprehensive analysis, Philadelphia, 1983, Davis.

Northrip JW, Logan GA, McKinney WC: Analysis of sport motion: anatomic and biomechanic perspectives, ed 3, Dubuque, Ia, 1983, Brown.

Piscopo J, Baley J: Kinesiology:the science of movement, New York, 1981, John Wiley & Sons.

Rasch PJ: Kinesiology and applied anatomy, ed 7, Philadelphia, 1989, Lea & Febiger.

*Royal Canadian Air Force exercise plans for physical fitness; XBX-Women, 5BX-Men, Mt Vernon, NY, 1962.

Scott MG: Analysis of human motion, ed 2, New York, 1963, Appleton-Century-Crofts.

Weineck J: Functional anatomy in sports, ed 2, St. Louis, 1990, Mosby.

Wells KF, Luttgens K: Kinesiology, ed . 7, Philadelphia, 1982, Saunders.

Wirhed R: Athletic ability and the anatomy of motion, London, 1984, Wolfe.

Zarins B, Andrews JR, Carson WG: Injuries to the throwing arm, Philadelphia, 1985, Saunders.

*Information on conditioning exercises.

Glossary

abduction Lateral movement away from the midline of the trunk, as in raising the arms or legs to the side horizontally.

acceleration The rate of change in velocity.

adduction Movement medially toward the midline of the trunk, as in lowering the arms to the side or legs back to the anatomical position.

agonist A muscle or muscle group that is described as being primarily responsible for a specific joint movement when contracting.

anatomical position The position of reference in which the subject is in the standing position, with feet together and palms of hands facing forward.

angle of pull The angle between the muscle insertion and the bone on which it inserts.

angular motion Motion involving rotation around an axis.

antagonist A muscle or muscle group that counteracts or opposes the contraction of another muscle or muscle group.

arthrodial joints Joints in which bones glide on each other in limited movement, as in the bones of the wrist (carpal) or bones of the foot (tarsal).

balance The ability to control equilibrium, either static or dynamic.

center of gravity The point at which all of body's mass and weight are equally balanced or equally distributed in all directions.

circumduction Circular movement of a bone at the joint, as in movement of the hip, shoulder, or trunk around a fixed point.

concentric contraction A contraction in which there is a shortening of the muscle.

condyloid joint Type of joint in which the bones permit movement in two planes without rotation, as in the wrist between the radius and the proximal row of the carpal bones or the second, third, fourth, and fifth metacarpophalangeal joints.

depression Inferior movement of the shoulder girdle, as in returning to the normal position from a shoulder shrug.

diagonal abduction Movement by a limb through a diagonal plane away from the midline of the body.

diagonal adduction Movement by a limb through a diagonal plane toward and across the midline of the body.

distal Farthest from the midline or point of reference; the hand is the most distal part of the upper extremity.

dorsal flexion Flexion movement of the ankle resulting in the top of foot moving toward the anterior tibia bone.

eccentric contraction Contraction in which there is lengthening of a muscle as a result of the force of gravity or a greater force than the contractile force.

elevation Superior movement of the shoulder girdle, as in shrugging the shoulders.

enarthrodial joint Type of joint which permits movement in all planes, as in the shoulder (glenohumeral) and hip joints.

equilibrium State of zero acceleration in which there is no change in the speed or direction of the body.

eversion Turning the sole of the foot outward or laterally, as in standing with the weight on the inner edge of the foot.

extension Straightening movement resulting in an increase of the angle in a joint by moving bones apart, as when the hand moves away from shoulder.

external rotation Rotary movement around the longitudinal axis of a bone away from the midline of the body. Also known as rotation laterally, outward rotation, and lateral rotation.

fascia Fibrous membrane covering, supporting, connecting, and separating muscles.

first-class lever A lever in which the axis (fulcrum) is between the force and the resistance, as in the extension of the elbow joint.

flexion Movement of the bones toward each other at a joint by decreasing the angle, as at the elbow or knee joint

force arm The distance between the axis and the point of force application.

ginglymus joint Type of joint which permits a wide range of movement in only one plane such as in the elbow, ankle, and knee joints.

hamstrings A common name given to the group of posterior thigh muscles: biceps femoris, semitendinosus, and semimembranosus.

horizontal abduction Movement of the humerus in the horizontal plane away from the midline of the body.

horizontal adduction Movement of the humerus in the horizontal plane toward the midline of the body.

insertion The point of attachment of a muscle farthest from the midline or center of the body.

internal rotation Rotary movement around the longitudinal axis of a bone toward the midline of the body. Also known as rotation medially, inward rotation, and medial rotation.

intrinsic muscles Muscles that are entirely contained within a specified body part; usually referring to the small, deep muscles found in the foot and hand.

inversion Turning the sole of the foot inward or medially, as in standing with the weight on the outer edge of the foot.

isokinetic Type of dynamic exercise usually using concentric and/or eccentric muscle contractions in which the speed (or velocity) of movement is constant and muscular contraction (usually maximal contraction) occurs throughout the movement.

isometric contraction A type of contraction with little or no shortening of the muscle resulting in no appreciable change in the joint angle.

isotonic Contraction occurring in which there is either shortening or lengthening in the muscle under tension; also known as a dynamic contraction and may be classified as being either concentric or eccentric.

kinesiology The science of movement, which includes anatomical (structural) and biomechanical (mechanical) aspects of movement.

lateral flexion Movement of the head and or trunk laterally away from the midline; abduction of spine.

lever A rigid bar (bone) that moves about an axis.

ligament A type of tough connective tissue that attaches bone to bone to provide static stability to joints.

linear motion Motion along a line.

opposition Diagonal movement of the thumb across the palmar surface of the hand to make contact with the fingers.

origin The point of attachment of a muscle closest to the midline or center of the body.

plantar flexion Extension movement of the ankle resulting in the foot and or toes moving away from the body.

pronation Internally rotating the radius to where it lies diagonally across the ulna, resulting in the palm-down position of the forearm; also used in referring to the combined movements of eversion, abduction, and external rotation of the foot and ankle.

protraction Forward movement of the shoulder girdle away from the spine; abduction of the scapula.

proximal Nearest to the midline or point of reference, the first digit of the hand or foot is proximal to the metatarsal.

quadriceps A common name given to the four muscles of the anterior aspect of the thigh: rectus femoris, vastus medialis, vastus intermedius, and vastus lateralis.

radial flexion Abduction movement at the wrist of the thumb side of the hand toward the forearm.

reduction Return of the spinal column to the anatomic position from lateral flexion; spine adduction.

resistance arm The distance between the axis and the point of resistance application.

retraction Backward movement of the shoulder girdle toward the spine; adduction of the scapula.

rotation Movement around the axis of a bone, such as the turning inward, outward, downward, or upward of a bone.

second-class lever A lever in which the resistance is between the axis (fulcrum) and the force (effort), as in plantar flexing the foot to raise up on the toes.

sellar joints Type of reciprocal reception that is found only in the thumb at the carpometacarpal joint and permits ball-and-socket movement, with the exception of rotation.

stability The resistance to a change in the body's acceleration; the resistance to a disturbance of the body's equilibrium.

supination Externally rotating the radius to where it lies parallel to the ulna, resulting in the palm-up position of the forearm; also used in referring to the combined movements of inversion, adduction, and internal rotation of the foot and ankle.

syndesmosis joint Type of joint held together by strong ligamentous structures that allow minimal movement between the bones such as the coracoclavicular joint and the inferior tibiofibular joint.

synchondrosis joint Type of joint separated by a fibrocartilage that allows very slight movement between the bones such as the symphysis pubis and the costochondral joints of the ribs with the sternum.

tendon Fibrous connective tissue, often cordlike in appearance, that connects muscles to bones and other structures.

third-class lever A lever in which the force (effort) is between the axis (fulcrum) and the resistance, as in flexion of the elbow joint.

trochoidal joint Type of joint with a rotational movement around a long axis, as in rotation of the radius at the radioulnar joint.

Ulnar flexion Adduction movement at the wrist of the little finger side of the hand toward the forearm.

Illustration credits

Page ii Ron Carlberg.

Chapter 1 1-1, through 1-3, Ernest W. Beck.

Chapter 2 2-1, 2-2, Linda Kimbrough; 2-3, John Hood; 2-4 through 2-8, Ernest W. Beck.

Chapter 3 3-1, Linda Kimbrough; 3-2, 3-3, John Hood; 3-4, Ernest W. Beck; 3-5, John Hood; 3-6 through 3-15, Ernest W. Beck.

Chapter 4 4-1 A-C, Linda Kimbrough; 4-2 A-D, 4-3 A, John Hood; 4-3 B, Ernest W. Beck; 4-4 A, John Hood; 4-4 B through 4-12, Ernest W. Beck.

Chapter 5 5-1, Ernest W. Beck; 5-2 A-F, John Hood; 5-3 through 5-7, 5-9 through 5-12, 5-15, Ernest W. Beck.

Chapter 6 6-1 A-B, John Hood; 6-2 A-C, 6-3 A-B, 6-4 A-B, Ron Carlberg.

Chapter 7 7-1, 7-3, Ernest W. Beck; 7-4 A-F, 7-5 A-D, John Hood; 7-6 through 7-23, Ernest W. Beck.

Chapter 8 8-1 A-C, Ernest W. Beck; 8-2 A-D, John Hood; 8-3, Linda Kimbrough; 8-4, 8-5, 8-6, 8-8, Ernest W. Beck.

Chapter 9 9-1, 9-2, 9-4, Ernest W. Beck; 9-5 A-F, John Hood; 9-6 through 9-12, Ernest W. Beck; 9-13, Linda Kimbrough; 9-14 through 9-17, Ernest W. Beck.

Chapter 10 10-1, Ernest W. Beck; 10-2 A-D, Linda Kimbrough; 10-2 E-F, Ernest W. Beck; 10-3 A-H, John Hood; 10-4 through 10-8, Ernest W. Beck; 10-9 A-C, Linda Kimbrough; 10-10, 10-11, Ernest W. Beck; 10-12 A-B, Linda Kimbrough.

Chapter 11 11-1 A-B, 11-2 A-B, John Hood; 11-4, Courtesy Universal Athletic Sales Co., Inc., Fresno, California; 11-6, 11-7 A-B, 11-8 A-B, Ron Carlberg.

(Note: There are no credits for chapter 12.)

Index

Page numbers in italics indicate illustration only.

Worksheets

CHAPTER ONE
Worksheet No. 1
On the posterior skeletal worksheet, list the names of the bones and all of the prominent features of each bone.

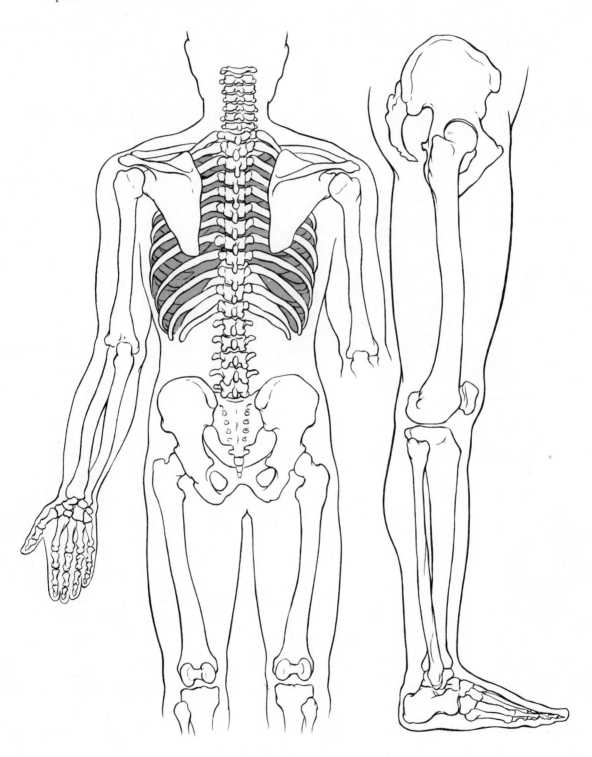

Worksheet No. 2
On the anterior skeletal worksheet, list the names of the bones and all of the prominent features of each bone.

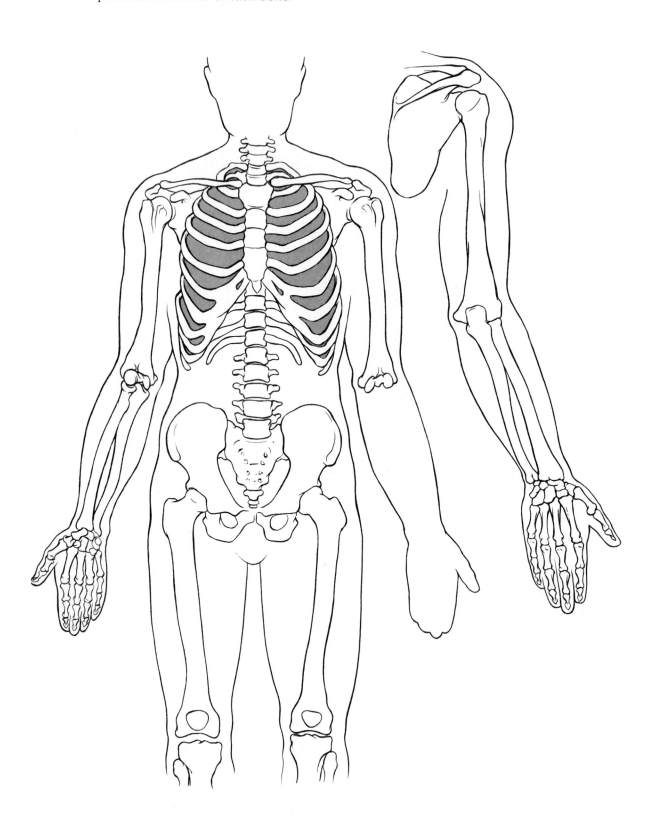

CHAPTER TWO

Worksheet No. 1

Draw and label on the worksheet the following listed muscles.

a. Trapezius
b. Rhomboid
c. Serratus anterior
d. Levator scapulae
e. Pectoralis minor

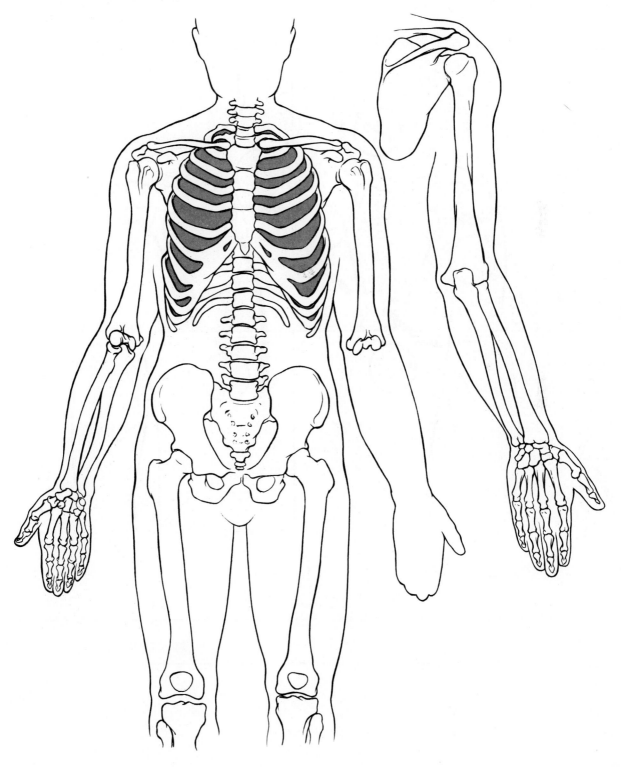

Worksheet No. 2

Label and indicate by arrows the following movements of the shoulder girdle.

a. Adduction
b. Abduction
c. Upward rotation
d. Downward rotation
e. Elevation
f. Depression

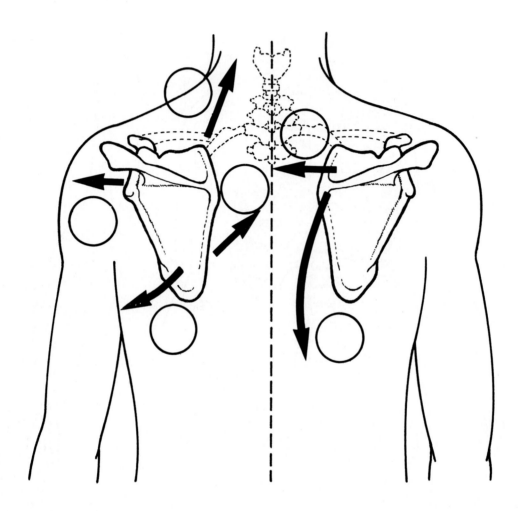

CHAPTER THREE

Worksheet No. 1

Draw and label on the worksheet the following muscles:

a. Deltoid
b. Supraspinatus
c. Subscapularis
d. Teres major
e. Infraspinatus
f. Teres minor
g. Latissimus dorsi
h. Pectoralis major
i. Coracobrachialis

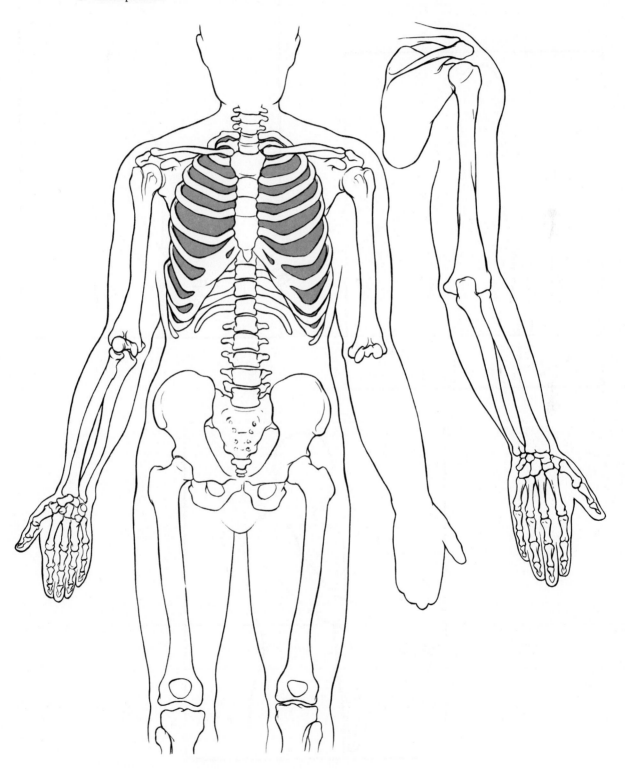

CHAPTER THREE

Worksheet No. 2

Label and indicate by arrows the following listed movements of the shoulder joint:

a. Abduction
b. Adduction
c. Flexion
d. Extension
e. Horizontal adduction
f. Horizontal abduction

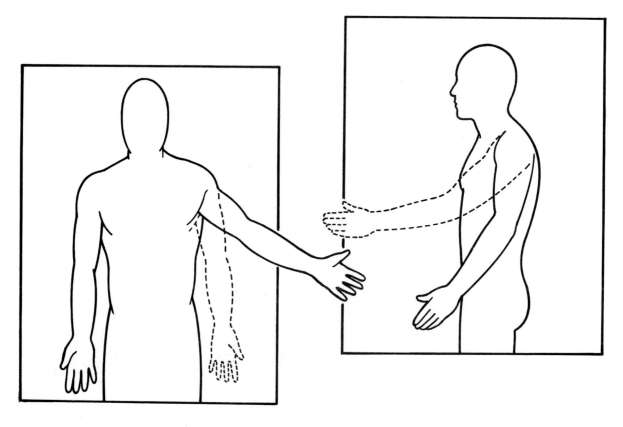

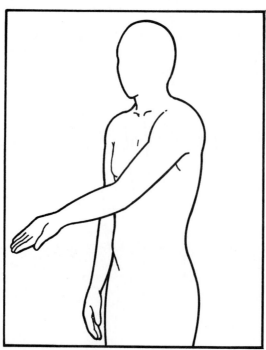

CHAPTER FOUR

Worksheet No. 1

Draw and label on the worksheet the following muscles:

a. Biceps brachii
b. Brachioradialis
c. Brachialis
d. Pronator teres

e. Supinator
f. Triceps brachii
g. Anconeus
h. Pronator quadratus

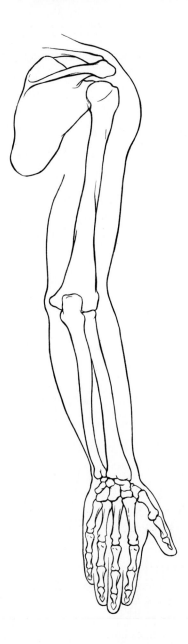
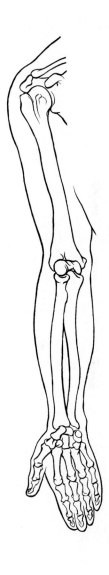

CHAPTER FIVE

Worksheet No. 1

Draw and label on the worksheet the following muscles.

a. Flexor pollicis longus
b. Flexor carpi radialis
c. Flexor carpi ulnaris
d. Extensor digitorum
e. Extensor pollicis longus
f. Extensor pollicis brevis
g. Extensor carpi ulnaris
h. Palmaris longus
i. Extensor carpi radialis longus
j. Extensor carpi radialis brevis
k. Extensor digit minimi
l. Extensor digitorum indicis
m. Flexor digitorum superficialis
n. Flexor digitorum profundus
o. Abductor pollicis longus

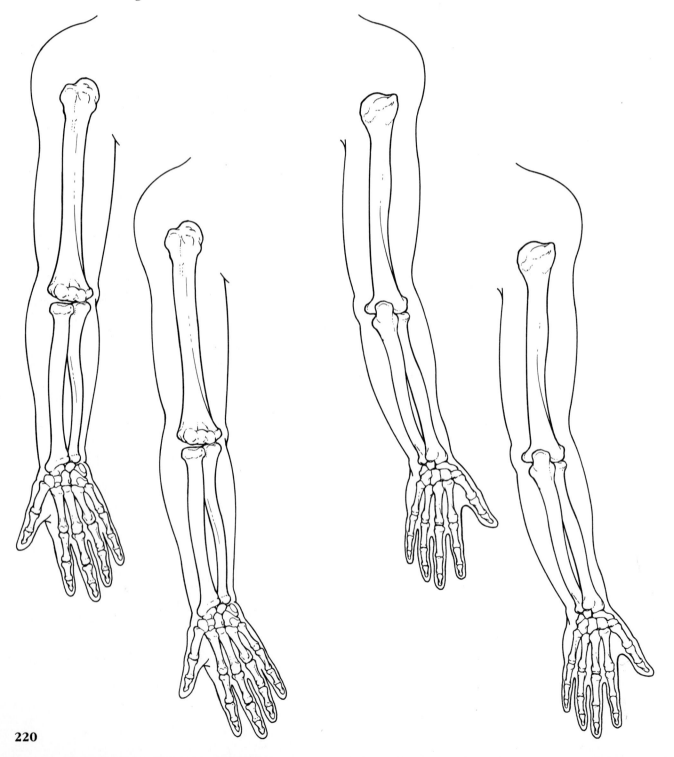

CHAPTER FIVE
Worksheet No. 2
Label and indicate by arrows the following movements of the radioulnar joint and wrist and hands:

Radioulnar joint	Wrist and hands
Pronation	Extension
Supination	Flexion

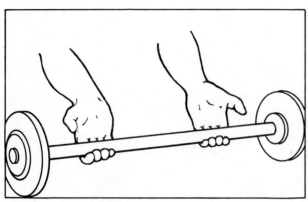
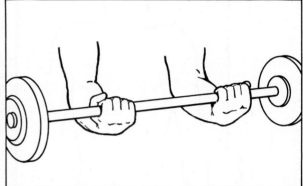

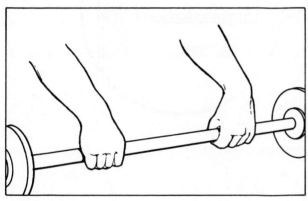
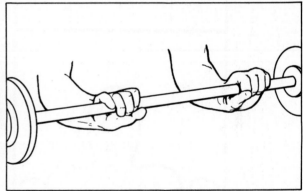

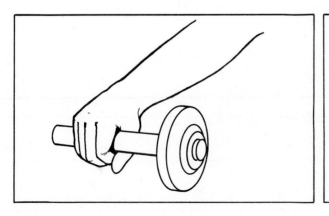
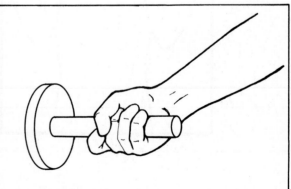

CHAPTER SIX

Worksheet No. 1

Analyze this exercise following the procedures explained in this chapter that include joint movement and muscles that produce these movements.

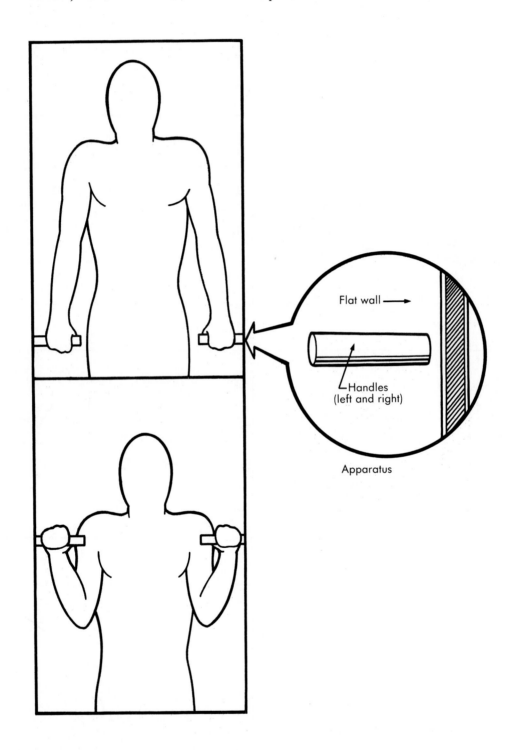

Flat wall →

Handles
(left and right)

Apparatus

Worksheet No. 1
Draw and label on the worksheet the anterior hip joint and pelvic girdle muscles.

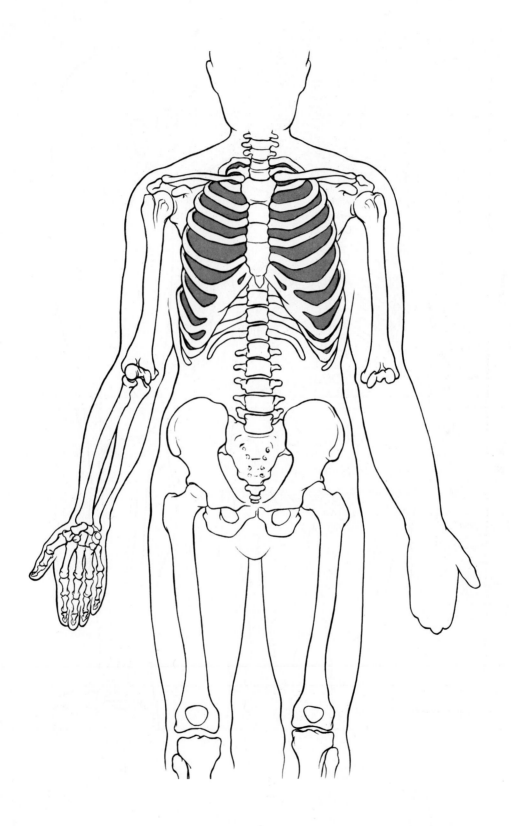

CHAPTER SEVEN
Worksheet No. 2
Draw and label on the worksheet the posterior hip and pelvic girdle muscles.

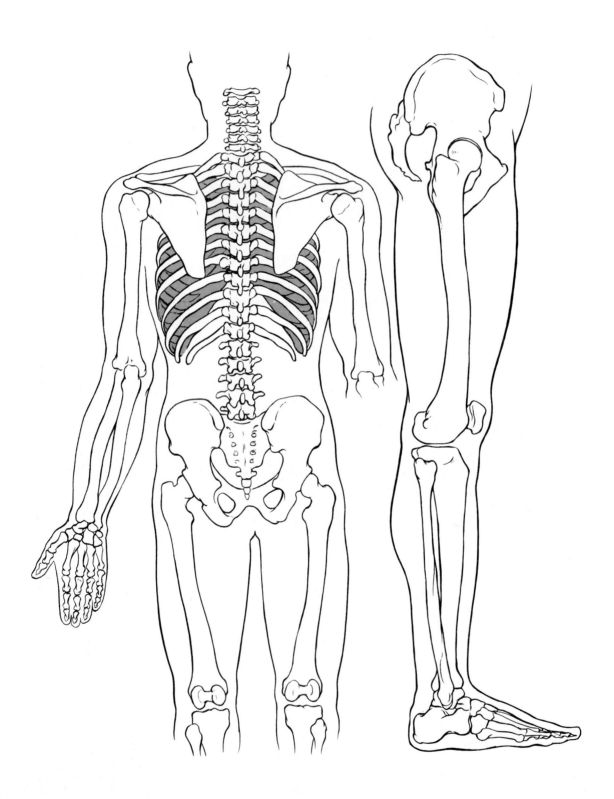

CHAPTER EIGHT
Worksheet No. 1
Draw and label on the worksheet the knee joint muscles.

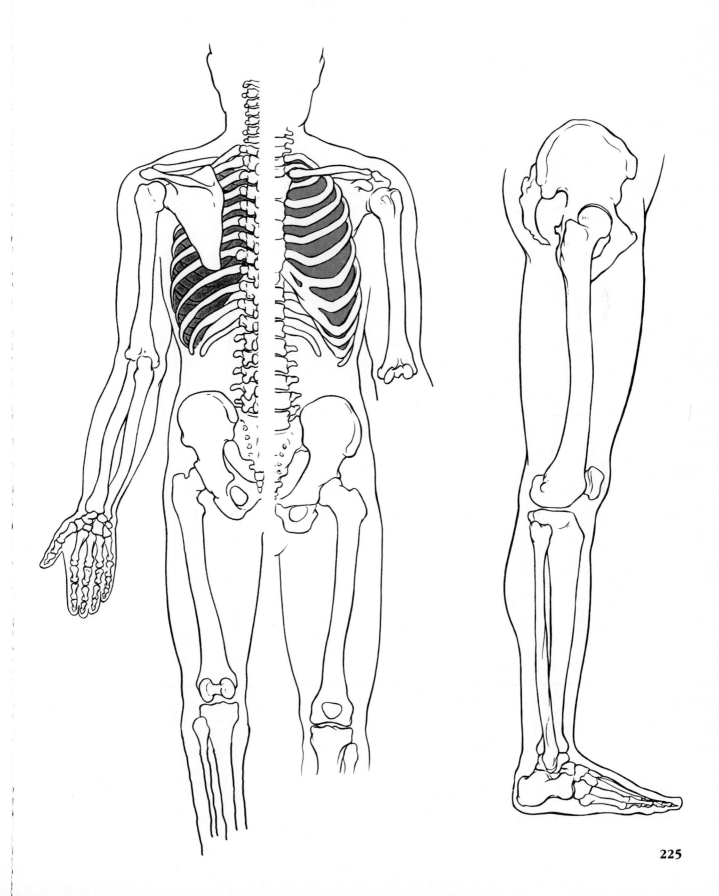

CHAPTER NINE

Worksheet No. 1

Draw and label on the worksheet the following muscles of the ankle and foot.

a. Tibialis anterior
b. Extensor digitorum longus
c. Peroneus longus
d. Peroneus brevis
e. Soleus
f. Peroneus tertius

g. Gastrocnemius
h. Extensor hallucis longus
i. Tibialis posterior
j. Flexor digitorum longus
k. Flexor hallucis longus

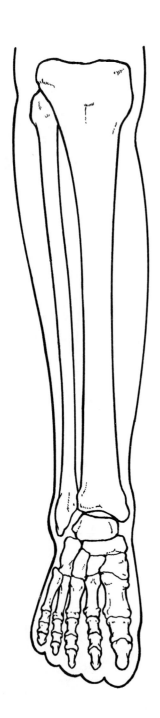
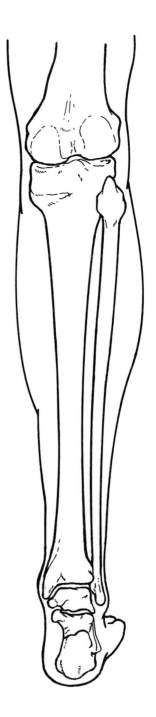

CHAPTER TEN
Worksheet No. 1
Draw and label the following muscles on the skeletal chart.

a. Rectus abdominis

b. External oblique abdominal

c. Internal oblique abdominal

d. Sternocleidomastoid

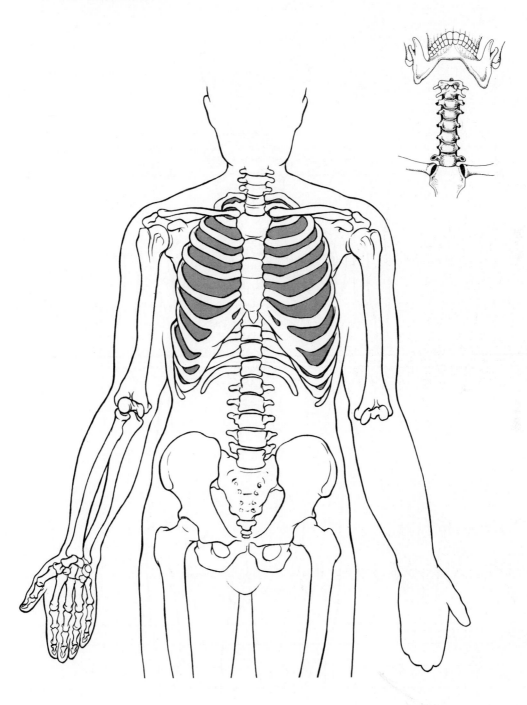

CHAPTER TEN
Worksheet No. 2
Draw and label the following muscles on the skeletal chart.
a. Erector spinae
b. Quadratus lumborum
c. Splenius-cervicis and capitis

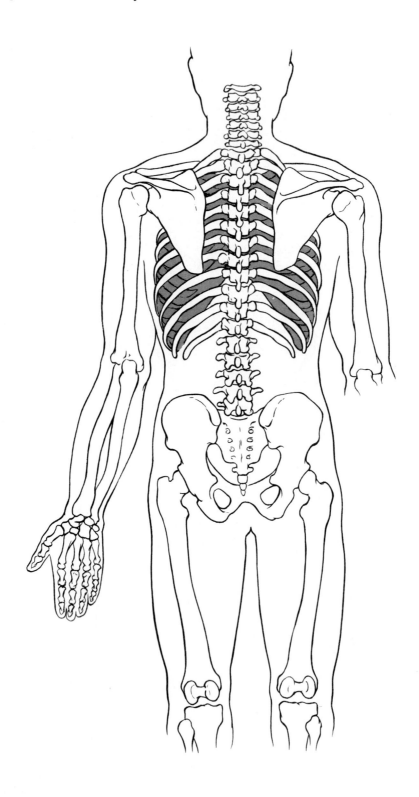